Acute Coronary Syndromes in Clinical Practice

Anthony A. Bavry and Deepak L. Bhatt
Editors

Acute Coronary Syndromes in Clinical Practice

 Springer

Editors

Anthony A. Bavry
Assistant Professor of Medicine
Division of Cardiovascular
    Medicine
University of Florida
FL, USA

Deepak L. Bhatt
Chief of Cardiology, VA Boston
Director, Interventional Program
VA Boston and Brigham and
    Women's Hospital
MA, USA

ISBN: 978-1-84800-357-6   e-ISBN: 978-1-84800-358-3
DOI 10.1007/978-1-84800-358-3

British Library Cataloguing in Publication Data
A catalogue record for this book is available from the British Library

Library of Congress Control Number: 2008938259

Printed on acid-free paper

Springer Science+Business Media
springer.com

To the interventional fellows I have worked with: Drs Chacko, Chhatriwalla, Christofferson, de Oliveiro, Duffy, Filby, Jefferson, Karha, Kelly, Overly, Rajagopal, Shishehbor, and Simpfendorfer. I am honored to have trained with such an exceptionally talented group of individuals.

AAB

To my wife Shanthala and to my sons Vinayak, Arjun, and Ram, for allowing me to spend time at the hospital caring for patients with acute coronary syndromes and at home writing about acute coronary syndromes.

DLB

Contents

Author biographies   ix
Preface   xi

1.   **Definition, epidemiology and prognosis**   **1**
   References   9

2.   **Pathophysiology**   **11**
   Atherosclerosis   11
   Plaque rupture   11
   The coagulation cascade   14
   References   14

3.   **Clinical manifestations**   **15**
   Symptoms and signs   15
   Biomarkers   16
   Electrocardiogram   18
   Summary   21
   References   21

4.   **Risk stratification**   **23**
   Non-ST-elevation ACS risk models   24
   ST-elevation risk models   31
   Summary   34
   References   35

5.   **Anti-platelet therapy**   **37**
   Aspirin   37
   Clopidogrel   39
   Prasugrel   40
   Glycoprotein IIb/IIIa inhibitors   42
   References   45

6.   **Anti-thrombin therapy**   **49**
   Unfractionated heparin   49
   Low-molecular-weight heparin   51

Direct thrombin inhibitors 54
Factor Xa inhibitors 56
Summary 57
References 58

7.   Miscellaneous therapy **61**
Statins 61
Angiotensin-converting enzyme inhibitors 62
Beta-blockers 63
Calcium-channel blockers 65
Nitrates/novel anti-anginal agents 65
Summary 66
References 66

8.   Revascularization and reperfusion therapy **69**
Revascularization therapy 69
Reperfusion therapy 75
Summary 75
References 76

9.   Controversies and future approaches **79**
Facilitated percutaneous coronary intervention 79
Early invasive versus conservative management 80
Culprit-vessel versus multi-vessel intervention 82
Drug-eluting stents versus bare-metal stents 82
Future approaches 85
Summary 86
References 86

Appendix: ACC/AHA and ESC practice guidelines **89**
Definitions for guideline recommendations
and level of evidence 89
Early invasive therapy versus conservative management 90
Adjunctive anti-platelet, anti-coagulation, medical therapies,
and risk stratisfication – invasive strategy 91
Adjunctive anti-platelet, anti-coagulation, medical therapies,
and risk stratisfication – conservative strategy 92

Index **95**

Author biographies

Anthony A Bavry MD, MPH, is an Assistant Professor of Medicine at the University of Florida. He received his medical degree from the University of Florida and a masters in public health from Harvard University. He completed his internal medicine residency at the University of Arizona, and general cardiology and interventional cardiology fellowship at the Cleveland Clinic.

Deepak L Bhatt MD, FACC, FSCAI, FESC, FACP, FCCP, FAHA, is Chief of Cardiology of the VA Boston Healthcare System and Director of the Integrated Interventional Cardiovascular Program at Brigham and Women's Hospital and the VA Boston Healthcare System. He is also a Senior Investigator in the TIMI Group and on the faculty of Harvard Medical School.

After graduating as valedictorian from the Boston Latin School, Dr Bhatt obtained his undergraduate science degree as a National Merit Scholar at the Massachusetts Institute of Technology, while also serving as a research associate at Harvard Medical School. He received his medical doctorate from Cornell University. His internship and residency in internal medicine were performed at the Hospital of the University of Pennsylvania, and his cardiovascular training was completed at the Cleveland Clinic. He also completed fellowships in interventional cardiology and cerebral and peripheral vascular intervention, as well as serving as chief interventional fellow at the Cleveland Clinic, where he went on to spend several years as an interventional cardiologist and Associate Professor of Medicine. He served for many years as the Director of the Interventional Cardiology Fellowship and as Associate Director of the Cardiovascular Medicine Fellowship. Dr Bhatt was listed in Best Doctors in America in 2005, 2006, 2007, and 2008.

Dr Bhatt's research interests include preventive cardiology, as well as the optimal management of patients with acute coronary syndromes. He also has research interests in advanced techniques in cardiac, cerebral, and peripheral intervention. He has authored or co-authored over 200 articles, including in *Circulation Research, Journal of the American Medical Association,*

Lancet, *Nature Reviews Drug Discovery*, and *New England Journal of Medicine*. He is on the editorial boards of *Acute Coronary Syndromes*, *American Heart Journal*, *Cardiosource* (Associate Editor, Clinical Trials), *CCI*, *Circulation*, *Indian Heart Journal*, *Journal of the American College of Cardiology* (named an Elite Reviewer in 2004, 2005, and 2006), and *Journal of Thrombosis and Thrombolysis*, and is Section Editor of Adjunctive Therapy for the *Journal of Invasive Cardiology*. He is the editor of *Essential Concepts in Cardiovascular Intervention* and *Guide to Peripheral and Cerebrovascular Intervention*, as well as co-editor of the *Handbook of Acute Coronary Syndromes*. He is the international principal investigator for the CHARISMA and CRESCENDO trials and co-principal investigator of the CHAMPION and LANCELOT trials. He serves as the co-chair of the REACH registry. He is also on the steering committees of ARCHIPELAGO, APPRAISE, ATLAS ACS-TIMI 46, CRUSADE, and SEPIA-PCI.

Dr Bhatt has been a visiting lecturer at a number of institutions, including Baylor College of Medicine, Boston University, Emory University, Massachusetts General Hospital/Harvard, Mayo Clinic, Penn State, University of Alabama, University of Massachusetts, University of North Carolina, University of Pennsylvania, University of Virginia, and Yale. He has also lectured internationally, including at the Brazilian Society of Cardiology, French Society of Cardiology, Japanese Society of Thrombosis and Hemostasis, Italian Society of Cardiology, Indonesian Heart Association, McGill University, McMaster University, Montreal Heart Institute, and Swiss Cardiac Society. He has been interviewed extensively by news agencies such as CBS, CNN, FOX, NBC, the *New York Times*, NPR, and the *Wall Street Journal* on topics ranging from premature coronary artery disease to the role of inflammation and genetics in heart attacks.

Preface

Acute coronary syndromes affect millions of individuals annually by causing considerable morbidity and mortality. In developed countries this disease remains the number one killer, despite significant improvements in its management over the last several decades. Acute coronary syndromes are challenging, as the field is a fast moving one with a rapid proliferation of drug and device trials. These new studies become incorporated into separate guideline recommendations by both American and European writing committees, which are frequently updated. Moreover, there are separate guideline recommendations for stable angina, non-ST-elevation acute coronary syndrome, ST-elevation myocardial infarction, and percutaneous coronary intervention. This may make it relatively difficult for practitioners to keep up-to-date with the field. Unfortunately, there is often a gap between the guideline recommendations and the care that is delivered in the 'real world.'

In this book we have attempted to distil the considerable literature on this topic into an accurate, succinct and up-to-date review of acute coronary syndromes. Many specialties are involved in the diagnosis and management of these syndromes; therefore, our audience includes a variety of practitioners: cardiologists, general practitioners, emergency medicine physicians, nurses, nurse practitioners, nursing students, physician trainees, medical students, pharmacists, and paramedics. We take the reader through the epidemiology and prognosis, diagnosis and clinical manifestations, risk stratification, and percutaneous and medical therapies across the entire spectrum of acute coronary syndromes. We end with a discussion on current controversies and future approaches to the treatment of acute coronary syndromes.

In short, we have taken pride and diligence in producing a review that we hope will provide our audience with the necessary knowledge to provide optimal evidence-based care for the acute coronary syndrome patient.

Anthony A Bavry
Deepak L Bhatt

Chapter 1

Definition, epidemiology, and prognosis

Cardiovascular disease is an all-encompassing term that includes diseases of the heart and coronary arteries, as well as diseases in other vascular beds. It is a major cause of death and disability in the United States, Europe, and worldwide (*see* Figure 1.1) [1]. Cardiovascular disease that is present in vascular beds outside of the coronary arteries is broadly termed peripheral arterial disease, and patients frequently have disease in such overlapping locations (*see* Figure 1.2) [2]. Examples include carotid and cerebrovascular disease, which are responsible for stroke and transient ischemic attack. Aortoiliac and femoral artery disease are responsible for limb ischemia and claudication. Cardiovascular disease can also manifest itself in stable or unstable forms. Stable coronary artery disease is characterized by stable angina or silent ischemia detected by stress testing, while unstable coronary artery disease (categorized, more generally, as coronary heart disease) includes myocardial infarction and unstable angina. An increasingly used and preferred term for an unstable event is acute coronary syndrome (ACS). ACS encompasses the spectrum from unstable angina to non-ST-elevation myocardial infarction and, finally, ST-elevation myocardial infarction. This

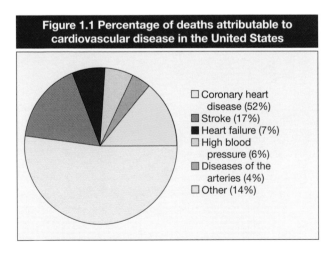

Figure 1.1 Percentage of deaths attributable to cardiovascular disease in the United States

☐ Coronary heart disease (52%)
■ Stroke (17%)
■ Heart failure (7%)
☐ High blood pressure (6%)
■ Diseases of the arteries (4%)
☐ Other (14%)

Reproduced with permission from the AHA [1].

A.A. Bavry, D.L. Bhatt (eds.), Acute Coronary Syndromes in Clinical Practice
DOI 10.1007/978-1-84800-358-3_1, © Springer-Verlag London Limited 2009

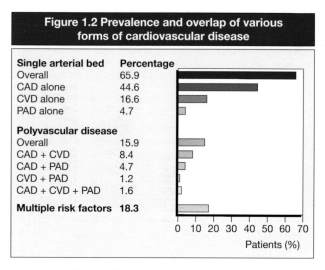

Figure 1.2 Prevalence and overlap of various forms of cardiovascular disease

Single arterial bed	Percentage
Overall	65.9
CAD alone	44.6
CVD alone	16.6
PAD alone	4.7
Polyvascular disease	
Overall	15.9
CAD + CVD	8.4
CAD + PAD	4.7
CVD + PAD	1.2
CAD + CVD + PAD	1.6
Multiple risk factors	**18.3**

CAD, coronary artery disease; CVD, cerebrovascular disease; PAD, peripheral arterial disease. Reproduced with permission from Bhatt *et al.* [2].

chapter will review the epidemiology and prognosis of cardiovascular disease in general, with a special focus on ACS.

In the United States, cardiovascular disease will affect nearly 80 million individuals at some point in their lives. Approximately one-half of these individuals are 65 years of age or older. In fact, the lifetime risk of cardiovascular disease is more than 70–80% (*see* Figure 1.3) [1]. Globally, approximately 10–15 million individuals die each year from cardiovascular disease, accounting for approximately one-third of all deaths [3,4]. The World Heath Organization (WHO) has projected that the number of deaths attributable to cardiovascular disease will continue to increase to the year 2030, while deaths from communicable causes will continue to decline [5].

There are nearly 8 million Americans who have had a myocardial infarction, with an incidence of approximately 1.5 million ACS per year and nearly 200,000 silent myocardial infarctions per year [1]. Of the ACS, two-thirds are due to unstable angina or non-ST-elevation myocardial infarction, while one-third is due to ST-elevation myocardial infarction. The incidence of ACS, similar to cardiovascular disease in general, increases with advanced

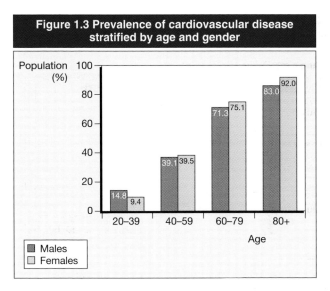

Figure 1.3 Prevalence of cardiovascular disease stratified by age and gender

Data include unstable coronary syndromes (myocardial infarction and unstable angina), heart failure, stroke and hypertension. Reproduced with permission from the AHA [1].

age, so that the mean age of first myocardial infarction is 66 years for men and 70 years for women. Globally, the WHO reported that deaths from cardiovascular diseases are highest for Finnish men and women from the United Kingdom [5].

ACS portends a poor prognosis. It is estimated that myocardial infarction results in 15 years of life lost to the individual, and translates into a 5-year mortality of 50% in patients greater than 70 years of age [1]. Data from a contemporary randomized clinical trial of patients admitted with a non-ST-elevation ACS found 30-day mortality to be 3% and death or myocardial infarction to be 14% [6]. Registry data also revealed the 30-day mortality for non-ST-elevation myocardial infarction to be 5.1%, which was similar to or slightly less than the mortality for ST-elevation myocardial infarction (5.1%), or ST-elevation myocardial infarction with reciprocal ST-depression (6.6%) [7]. In a nonselected population of patients with ST-elevation myocardial infarction undergoing lytic therapy, 30-day mortality may be as high as 10% [8]. Although early outcomes are similar across the ACS spectrum, patients with non-ST-elevation myocardial infarction have a higher late mortality (8.9% at 6 months), compared with ST-elevation myocardial infarction (6.8% at 6 months) [7]. Not surprisingly, cardiovascular disease is responsible for the most deaths in the United States at a rate of approximately one death every minute (*see* Figure 1.4) [1].

Although the burden of cardiovascular disease is tremendous, mortality from myocardial infarction has been declining for the last several decades after peaking in the early 1970s [9]. In the United States, the death rate from coronary heart disease in men declined from 540 deaths per 100,000 population to 267 deaths per 100,000 population during the period 1980–2000. In women, the death rate declined from 263 deaths per 100,000 population to 134 deaths per 100,000 population over the same time period [10]. It is estimated that approximately half of this reduction is attributable to improved cardiovascular treatments. Examples in acute myocardial infarction include the use of cardiopulmonary resuscitation, aspirin, beta-blockers, angiotensin-converting enzyme (ACE) inhibitors, thrombolysis, and primary angioplasty. The use of angioplasty has increased dramatically, although the utilization of this therapy is still far from optimal among eligible individuals [11]. The other half of the reduction in mortality is attributable to cardiovas-

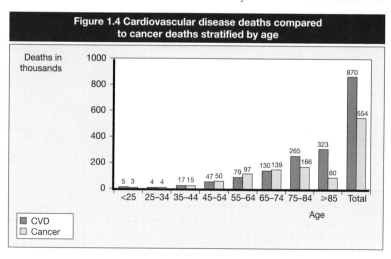

Figure 1.4 Cardiovascular disease deaths compared to cancer deaths stratified by age

CVD, cardiovascular disease. Reproduced with permission from the AHA [1].

cular risk factor modification. From 1980 to 2000, the prevalence of smoking and physical inactivity was reduced by 32% and 8%, respectively. Systolic blood pressure was reduced by an absolute of 4 mmHg and total cholesterol declined by an absolute of 6 mmol/L. The change in risk factors may have also changed the landscape of ACS since there are now proportionately more non-ST ACS relative to ST-elevation events [12]. Unfortunately, part of this benefit has been offset by increases in diabetes and body mass index. Moreover, the population-wide decline in modifiable risk factors is likely attenuated due to the global underutilization of anti-hypertensive and statin medications [2]. A reduction in coronary mortality has also been documented in other developed countries such as England and Wales [13], Finland [14], and the Netherlands [15]. While this is reassuring, the reality is that more people are living longer with cardiovascular disease after having suffered an acute event [16].

The GRACE (Global Registry of Acute Coronary Events) registry tracks detailed information including cardiovascular outcomes across the spectrum of ACS [17]. From 1999 to 2006 the use of guideline-recommended medications increased among non-ST-elevation myocardial infarction (see Figure 1.5) and ST-elevation myocardial infarction (see Figure 1.6). The proportion of patients who did not receive any form of revascularization therapy for non-ST-elevation ACS decreased from 69% to 58% ($p<0.001$) due to a significant increase in the use of percutaneous coronary intervention (from 17% to 35%; $p<0.001$). In ST-elevation myocardial infarction, the use of mechanical reperfusion increased from 32% to 64%, while pharmacological reperfusion decreased from 50% to 28%; therefore, the proportion of patients that did not receive any reperfusion therapy remained constant at approximately one-third. Over this follow-up period, early and late death, early myocardial infarction and late stroke were reduced among non-ST-elevation myocardial infarction patients, while, in-hospital death, cardiogenic shock, myocardial infarction and late stroke were reduced among ST-elevation myocardial infarction patients.

In summary, cardiovascular disease, especially ACS, represents one of the most significant public health priorities across the globe. In the last several decades, improvements have been made in reducing the prevalence of smoking and hypertension, although unfortunately obesity and diabetes have increased during this time. As a result of the change in risk factors, the proportion of ST-elevation myocardial infarction has declined relative

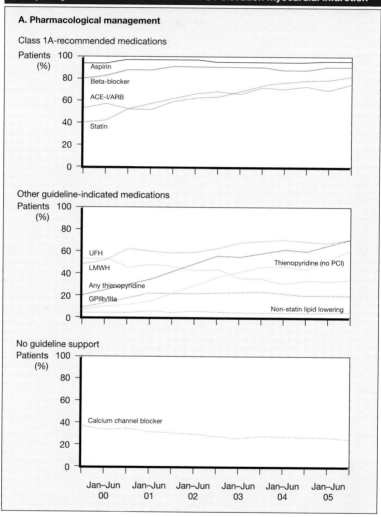

Figure 1.5 The use of guideline-recommended therapies and frequency of revascularization for non-ST-elevation myocardial infarction

ACE-I, angiotensin-converting enzyme inhibitor; ARB, angiotensin II receptor blocker; GP, glycoprotein; LMWH, low-molecular-weight heparin; PCI, percutaneous coronary intervention; UFH, unfractionated heparin. Reproduced with permission from Fox *et al.* [17].

Figure 1.5 *Continued*. The use of guideline-recommended therapies and frequency of revascularization for non-ST-elevation myocardial infarction

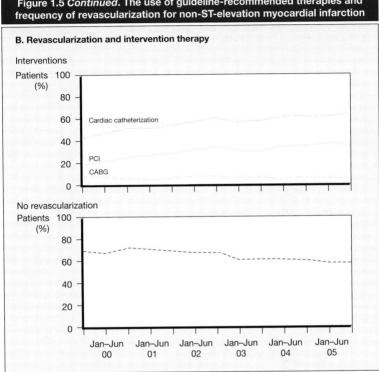

CABG, coronary artery bypass graft; PCI, percutaneous coronary intervention.
Reproduced with permission from Fox *et al.* [17].

to non-ST-elevation ACS. While this is good, the long-term prognosis of non-ST-elevation ACS remains poor. The last several decades have also seen improvements in reperfusion, revascularization, and adjuvant medical therapies, which have translated into decreased case-fatality for acute myocardial infarction. Thus, while we can applaud the significant achievements that have taken place, there is much room for improvement in the care of ACS patients.

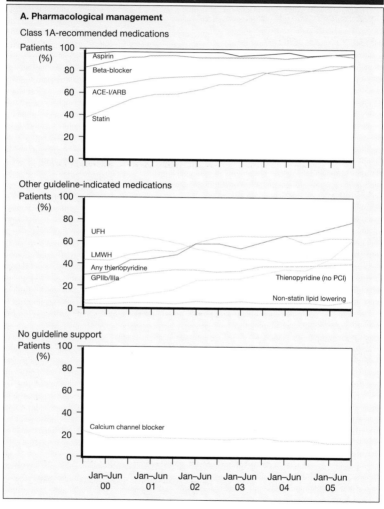

Figure 1.6 The use of guideline-recommended therapies and frequency of mechanical or pharmacological reperfusion for ST-elevation myocardial infarction

ACE-I, angiotensin-converting enzyme inhibitor; ARB, angiotensin II receptor blocker; GP, glycoprotein; LMWH, low-molecular-weight heparin; PCI, percutaneous coronary intervention; UFH, unfractionated heparin. Reproduced with permission from Fox *et al.* [17].

Figure 1.6 *Continued*. The use of guideline-recommended therapies and frequency of mechanical or pharmacological reperfusion for ST-elevation myocardial infarction

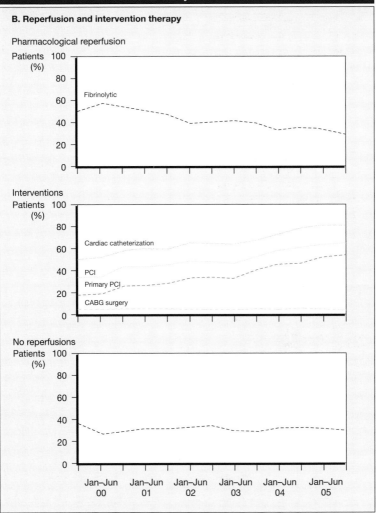

B. Reperfusion and intervention therapy

CABG, coronary artery bypass graft; PCI, percutaneous coronary intervention.
Reproduced with permission from Fox *et al.* [17].

References

1.   American Heart Association. Heart disease and stroke statistics – 2008 update at-a-glance. Available at: *www.americanheart.org/downloadable/heart/1200082005246HS_Stats%202008.final.pdf*. Last accessed January 2008.

2.   Bhatt DL, Steg PG, Ohman EM, *et al*. International prevalence, recognition, and treatment of cardiovascular risk factors in outpatients with atherothrombosis. *JAMA* 2006; **295**:180–189.

3.   American Heart Association. International cardiovascular disease statistics: statistical fact sheet – populations. 2007 update. Available at: *www.americanheart.org/downloadable/ heart/1177593979236FS06INTL07.pdf*. Last accessed December 2007.

4.   Murray CJ, Lopez AD. Mortality by cause for eight regions of the world: global burden of disease study. *Lancet* 1997; **349**:1269–1276.

5.   Mathers CD, Loncar D. Projections of global mortality and burden of disease from 2002 to 2030. *PLoS Med* 2006; **3**:e442.

6.   The SYNERGY Trial Investigators. Enoxaparin vs unfractionated heparin in high-risk patients with non-ST-segment elevation acute coronary syndromes managed with an intended early invasive strategy. Primary results of the SYNERGY randomized trial. *JAMA* 2004; **292**:45–54.

7.   Savonitto S, Ardissino D, Granger CB, *et al*. Prognostic value of the admission electrocardiogram in acute coronary syndromes. *JAMA* 1999; **281**:707–713.

8.   White HD. Thrombin-specific anticoagulation with bivalirudin versus heparin in patients receiving fibrinolytic therapy for acute myocardial infarction: the HERO-2 randomized trial. *Lancet* 2001; **358**:1855–1863.

9.   Fuster V. Epidemic of cardiovascular disease and stroke: the three main challenges. Presented at the 71st Scientific Sessions of the American Heart Association. *Circulation* 1999; **99**:1132–1137.

10.   Ford ES, Ajani UA, Croft JB, *et al*. Explaining the decrease in U.S. deaths from coronary disease, 1980–200. *N Engl J Med* 2007; **356**:2388–2398.

11.   Bhatt DL, Roe MT, Peterson ED, *et al*. Utilization of early invasive management strategies for high-risk patients with non-ST-segment elevation acute coronary syndromes. Results from the CRUSADE quality improvement initiative. *JAMA* 2004; **292**:2096–2104.

12.   Rogers WJ, Canto JG, Lambrew CT, *et al*. Temporal trends in the treatment of over 1.5 million patients with myocardial infarction in the U.S. from 1990 through 1999: the National Registry of Myocardial Infarction 1, 2 and 3. *J Am Coll Cardiol* 2000; **36**:2056–2063.

13.   Unal B, Critchley A, Capewell S. Explaining the decline in coronary heart disease mortality in England and Wales between 1981 and 2000. *Circulation* 2004; **109**:1101–1107.

14.   Laatikainen T, Critchley J, Vartiainen E, *et al*. Explaining the decline in coronary heart disease mortality in Finland between 1982 and 1997. *Am J Epidemiol* 2005; **162**:764–773.

15.   Bots ML, Grobbee DE. Decline of coronary heart disease mortality in the Netherlands from 1978 to 1985: contribution of medical care and changes over time in presence of major cardiovascular risk factors. *J Cardiovasc Risk* 1996; **3**:271–276.

16.   Lenfant C. Heart research: celebration and renewal. *Circulation* 1997; **96**:3822–3823.

17.   Fox KAA, Steg PG, Eagle KA, *et al*.; for the GRACE Investigators. Decline in rates of death and heart failure in acute coronary syndromes, 1999–2006. *JAMA* 2007; **297**:1892–1900.

Chapter 2

Pathophysiology

This chapter reviews the key elements in the pathophysiology and natural history of atherosclerosis. The interaction between the coagulation cascade and platelet physiology will also be discussed. Our understanding of the complex pathophysiology of atherosclerosis, the coagulation cascade, and platelet physiology is important in order to optimize pharmaceutical and device therapy.

Atherosclerosis

The development of atherosclerosis is influenced by an individual's risk factors: hypertension, hyperlipidemia, diabetes, and smoking. Atherosclerosis progresses over many decades until it is clinically detected [1]. Intimal thickening is present early in life; however, this is not felt to be pathologic. In the second to third decade of life, monocytes infiltrate the subintima. Once in the subintima, monocytes become macrophages, which become foam cells upon the ingestion of cholesterol. This is called a fatty streak or fatty dot and occurs early in the atherosclerotic disease process, although it progresses to an advanced plaque as a necrotic core develops. Expansion of this lipid content into a necrotic core occurs along with degradation of the extracellular matrix by matrix metalloproteinases and other inflammatory cytokines. Hemorrhage from the vasa vasorum may also contribute to the enlargement of the necrotic core. This process is more likely to occur at arterial branch points, which are areas of low shear stress. At this point, a vulnerable plaque may be present, characterized by a large necrotic lipid core underlying a thin fibrous cap. This is also referred to as a thin cap fibroatheroma and it is prone to rupture at its shoulder. The thin fibrous cap is composed of macrophages, lymphocytes, type I collagen, and relatively few smooth muscle cells [2].

Plaque rupture

Plaque rupture is responsible for most causes of sudden death and acute coronary syndromes [3]. Microscopically, plaques that rupture have decreased smooth muscle cells and increased macrophages and inflammatory cells. Macroscopically, vulnerable plaques are usually characterized by expansion of the external elastic media, referred to as positive remodeling,

A.A. Bavry, D.L. Bhatt (eds.), Acute Coronary Syndromes in Clinical Practice
DOI 10.1007/978-1-84800-358-3_2, © Springer-Verlag London Limited 2009

which preserves the luminal area. This is in contrast to patients with stable coronary artery disease who usually display negative remodeling or luminal narrowing. A rupture that leads to coronary occlusion is termed a ST-elevation myocardial infarction, while partial occlusion is a non-ST-elevation acute coronary syndrome (*see* Figure 2.1) [4]. Plaque rupture is more common in older individuals.

Recently, it has been discovered that vulnerable plaques can undergo frequent asymptomatic rupture with healing. Healing is characterized by

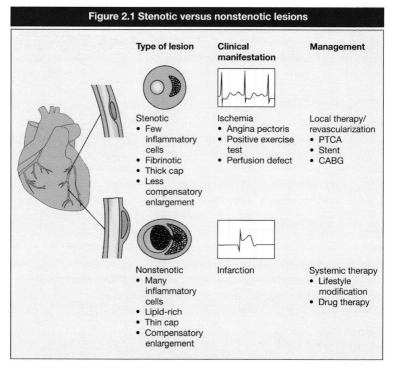

Figure 2.1 Stenotic versus nonstenotic lesions

Type of lesion	Clinical manifestation	Management
Stenotic • Few inflammatory cells • Fibrinotic • Thick cap • Less compensatory enlargement	Ischemia • Angina pectoris • Positive exercise test • Perfusion defect	Local therapy/revascularization • PTCA • Stent • CABG
Nonstenotic • Many inflammatory cells • Lipid-rich • Thin cap • Compensatory enlargement	Infarction	Systemic therapy • Lifestyle modification • Drug therapy

Stenotic lesions tend to be associated with thick fibrous caps and produce stable angina, while vulnerable plaques have a large lipid cores with thin caps and produce unstable coronary events. CABG, coronary artery bypass grafting; PTCA, percutaneous transluminal coronary angioplasty, Reprinted with permission from Libby & Theroux [4].

progressive thickening of the fibrous cap. While it is possible that each rupture can be subclinical, over time this process may result in luminal narrowing and cause stable angina [5]. An important finding is that most unstable coronary events originate from nonflow-limiting lesions (e.g., less than 70% stenosis) [6]. The implication is that revascularization of a severe coronary stenosis is usually done with the intent of symptom relief, rather than reduction in myocardial infarction or death. The next most common cause of unstable coronary events is plaque erosion, characterized by increased smooth muscle cells and decreased macrophages. Plaque erosion is frequently seen in younger individuals. The least common cause of an unstable coronary event is a calcified nodule (*see* Figure 2.2) [4].

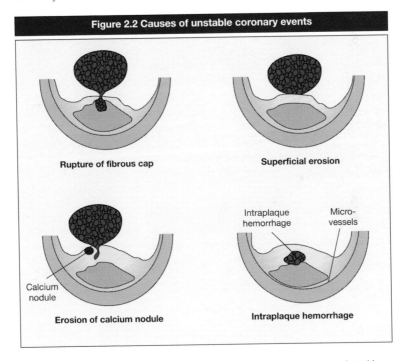

Figure 2.2 Causes of unstable coronary events

Rupture of fibrous cap

Superficial erosion

Calcium nodule

Erosion of calcium nodule

Intraplaque hemorrhage

Micro-vessels

Intraplaque hemorrhage

The most common cause of an unstable coronary event is rupture into a vulnerable plaque, although other mechanisms are possible. Reprinted with permission from Libby & Theroux [4].

The coagulation cascade

The coagulation cascade is accelerated on the surface of platelets. This process can be initiated from multiple points; however, binding of the platelet glycoprotein VI receptor to subendothelial collagen is one of the important steps after plaque rupture. This results in platelet adhesion to the subendothelium followed by platelet activation. Fibrinogen mediates the aggregation of activated platelets through the cross-linking of the glycoprotein IIb/IIIa receptor. This is called the final common pathway of platelet aggregation. Glycoprotein IIb/IIIa inhibitors act by preventing the binding of fibrinogen to this receptor. Aspirin blocks cyclooxygenase, which prevents the conversion of arachidonic acid to prostaglandin G_2 and thromboxane A_2. These two agents cause potent platelet aggregation and vasoconstriction. Thienopyridines (e.g., clopidogrel) prevent platelet activation and aggregation by blocking the platelet adenosine diphosphate receptor. Aggregated platelets combine with fibrin to form thrombus. A platelet-rich thrombus forms at areas of high shear stress and is called a white thrombus, while a fibrin-rich thrombus is called a red thrombus. A red thrombus forms at areas of relative hemostasis, and can therefore trap red blood cells within the fibrin mesh. Fibrin is the final product of the coagulation cascade, which is the meeting point of the extrinsic and intrinsic pathways. Exposure of tissue factor after plaque rupture initiates the process that converts prothrombin to thrombin, which in turn converts fibrinogen to fibrin. Tissue factor is the main stimulus for thrombin generation after plaque disruption.

References

1. Libby P. Molecular bases of the acute coronary syndromes. *Circulation* 1995; **91**:2844–2850.

2. Kolodgie FD, Burke AP, Farb A, *et al*. The thin-cap fibroatheroma: a type of vulnerable plaque: the major precursor lesion to acute coronary syndromes. *Curr Opin Cardiol* 2001; **16**:285–292.

3. Virmani R, Kolodgie FD, Burke AP, *et al*. Lessons from sudden coronary death: a comprehensive morphological classification scheme for atherosclerotic lesions. *Arterioscler Thromb Vasc Biol* 2000; **20**:1262–1275.

4. Libby P, Theroux P. Pathophysiology of Coronary Artery Disease. *Circulation* 2005; **111**:3481–3488.

5. Burke AP, Kolodgie FD, Farb A, *et al*. Healed plaque ruptures and sudden coronary death: evidence that subclinical rupture has a role in plaque progression. *Circulation* 2001; **103**:934–940.

6. Ambrose JA, Tannenbaum MA, Alexopoulos D, *et al*. Angiographic progression of coronary artery disease and the development of myocardial infarction. *J Am Coll Cardiol* 1988; **12**:56–62.

Chapter 3

Clinical manifestations

There is a short window of opportunity with ACS, where the prompt establishment of reperfusion therapy dramatically reduces left ventricular dysfunction and improves survival [1]. Accordingly, the initial aim with ACS is to expeditiously make the correct diagnosis. While this may seem overly simplistic, many patients are slow to seek medical attention or there is a long delay in establishing a correct diagnosis. Even when a correct diagnosis is made, delays may exist in bringing optimal therapy to patients who are most in need. Moreover, many patients who present to emergency departments with ACS are incorrectly diagnosed [2]. Attempts to diagnose every case of ACS can lead to excess false positive diagnoses with resultant high healthcare costs and unnecessary patient anxiety [3]. High-risk populations include late presenters, women, people with diabetes, and the elderly, where signs and symptoms of ACS may be protean [4]. Women with typical anginal symptoms and angiographically normal coronaries can still suffer from poor prognosis due to microvascular dysfunction [5]. Additionally, individuals presenting with left bundle branch block or paced rhythms, renal insufficiency, ACS within the peri-operative period and post-myocardial infarction angina are all important populations that require extra vigilance for adverse outcomes. This section will discuss the standard diagnosis of ACS that consists of signs and symptoms, biomarkers, and electrocardiograms, but will also focus on the special populations that need heightened awareness and the different strategies that can be used to make a prompt and accurate diagnosis.

Symptoms and signs

Traditionally, the diagnosis of ACS centers on symptoms, biomarkers and electrocardiograms. Symptoms are one of the most important means by which to make a diagnosis of ACS as they are usually the first opportunity to make the correct diagnosis and initiate prompt therapy. Unfortunately, this is also the area where misdiagnosis can cause a misappropriation of resources and result in poor outcomes. Therefore, it is important that practitioners have a good knowledge of ACS symptomatology [6]. The likelihood that anginal symptoms are attributable to obstructive coronary disease is increased in patients with prior coronary artery revascularization or previously documented coronary

A.A. Bavry, D.L. Bhatt (eds.), Acute Coronary Syndromes in Clinical Practice
DOI 10.1007/978-1-84800-358-3_3, © Springer-Verlag London Limited 2009

artery disease. Typical ACS symptoms are described as substernal chest heaviness, although there is great variation beyond this initial brief description that includes the location and quality of angina. Chest pain that is sharp, stabbing or pleuritic is uncommon, although it can be seen in some cases of ACS [7].

While the typical location is substernal, angina can often present on the left side of the chest, as well as partially or entirely in the neck, jaw, shoulder, arm, or back. These varied locations for angina can misdirect the diagnostic workup toward other considerations, including aortic dissection, pulmonary embolus, as well as less serious considerations such as costochondritis or musculoskeletal disorders. Moreover, some patients may present with silent or vague symptoms that can make establishing the correct diagnosis especially problematic. Silent or vague symptoms are usually seen in women, the elderly, and patients with diabetes; therefore, ACS should always be considered early in these groups. Relief of angina with administration of nitroglycerin is felt to increase the likelihood of the presence of obstructive coronary disease, although this agent can also improve noncardiac sources of chest pain [8].

Accompanied signs and symptoms of angina include dyspnea, nausea, diaphoresis, and anxiety, which are generally, although not universally, more common with ST-elevation myocardial infarction. With ST-elevation myocardial infarction, symptoms are not relieved with rest or nitroglycerin. Prompt resolution of ST elevation after administration of nitroglycerin is better categorized as non-ST-elevation myocardial infarction or ACS with transient ST-elevation. This should raise the suspicion of coronary spasm, but intermittent occlusion of a coronary artery instead of a persistent thrombotic occlusion is more likely. An important feature of unstable angina and non-ST-elevation myocardial infarction is that symptoms are new onset and usually present at rest unlike stable angina, where rest and/or nitroglycerin characteristically provide symptom relief. Angina that is exertional in nature may also be categorized as unstable if the symptoms represent a worsening from the patient's baseline [6].

Biomarkers

Biomarkers are important for firmly establishing an accurate diagnosis of ACS. They are also useful for risk stratification and prognostication, which can aid in determining the optimal therapy for a patient. Patients without elevated biomarkers and no other high-risk features can often be managed in a dedicated chest pain unit [9]. The most commonly used biomarkers include troponin I and T, as well as total creatine kinase (CK) and the myocardial band isoenzyme of CK (CK-MB) [10]. Troponin I and T become elevated 6 hours after ischemic injury, and can remain elevated for 2 weeks. Total and CK-MB isoenzyme become elevated 4–6 hours after ischemic injury and are especially useful for detecting re-infarction. Initially, troponin biomarkers were considered highly specific for ACS; however, various disease states and conditions can also elevate troponin levels (*see* Figure 3.1). A troponin level that is found to be elevated in a clinical context that is unlikely to be an ACS should be interpreted with caution. A common example is minimally elevated troponin in a patient with renal insufficiency in septic shock. In such a situation, minimally elevated troponin may not represent a true ACS, but it still portends a poor prognosis and merits aggressive risk factor modification [11]. In patients with renal insufficiency, CK values (total and CK-MB) can be especially useful for diagnosing and managing ACS. Elevated CK-MB levels in the absence of elevated total CK is associated with a poor prognosis [12]. Myoglobin is also sometimes used, although this biomarker suffers from even poorer specificity relative to the aforementioned enzymes. Therefore, myoglobin values are rarely used alone or in combination with CK and troponin values in making a diagnosis of ACS.

Figure 3.1 Conditions that can cause an elevation in troponin I or T values outside of ACS

Renal insufficiency

Pulmonary embolus

(Myo)pericarditis

Decompensated heart failure

Tako-tsubo syndrome

Coronary vasospasm

Critical illness, including extensive burns and sepsis

Cardiac contusion, trauma, and surgery

Electrical cardioversion/defibrillation

Electrophysiological procedures, including pulmonary vein isolation and arrhythmia ablation procedures

In ST-elevation myocardial infarction, biomarkers have less of an initial role since the working diagnosis is made by symptoms and electrocardiographic findings. In this population, biomarkers are important to gauge the size of an infarct and to risk stratify the patient after reperfusion. Waiting for cardiac biomarkers to return before making a diagnosis of ST-elevation myocardial infarction and starting reperfusion therapy is harmful and contraindicated. In contrast, cardiac biomarkers can help to risk stratify patients who present with chest pain of unclear etiology. Patients with positive biomarkers constitute a high-risk group relative to negative biomarker patients, and should receive appropriately aggressive therapy. By definition, cardiac biomarkers are negative in unstable angina patients, although dynamic and ischemic electrocardiographic changes should be present. Since unstable angina patients are a relatively high-risk group, in general they should receive the same therapy as non-ST-elevation myocardial infarction patients. A patient initially diagnosed with unstable angina based on symptoms and ischemic electrocardiographic findings, who is later found to have elevated biomarkers should be re-classified as non-ST-elevation myocardial infarction.

Electrocardiogram

The electrocardiogram is a central diagnostic test of cardiology since it is inexpensive, readily available, and provides quick and accurate information to risk stratify patients and direct therapy. However, important caveats to the electrocardiogram should be remembered, such as the differential diagnosis for ST-elevation (*see* Figure 3.2) [13]. Historically, myocardial infarctions were categorized as Q-wave or non-Q-wave events, which are terminal findings in a dynamic and evolving electrocardiographic process. Such an approach takes hours to days to make a diagnosis, at which time the window of opportunity to abort the myocardial infarction has largely passed. Presently, the electrocardiogram is used to rapidly triage patients into ST- or non-ST-elevation ACS pathways. This approach immediately risk stratifies patients and identifies those who urgently need reperfusion therapy. The electrocardiogram should be obtained early in patients who present with silent or vague symptoms. Nausea and fatigue in elderly patients with diabetes might be due to ACS and therefore needs to be diagnosed quickly. The electrocardiogram shows a spectrum of risk where combined ST elevation and depression represents the highest risk [14]. On the lower end of the spectrum are small inverted T-waves, while ST depres-

Figure 3.2 ST-segment elevation in normal circumstances and in various conditions

Condition	Features
Normal (so-called male pattern)	Elevation of 1–3 mm Most marked in V2 Concave Seen in approximately 90% of healthy young men; therefore, normal
Early repolarization	Most marked in V4, with notching at J-point Tall, upright T-waves Reciprocal ST depression in aVR, not in aVL, when limb leads are involved
ST elevation of normal variant	Seen in V3 through V5 with inverted T-waves Short QT, high QRS voltage
Left ventricular hypertrophy	Concave Other features of left ventricular hypertrophy
Left bundle branch block	Concave ST-segment deviation discordant from the QRS
Acute pericarditis	Diffuse ST-segment elevation Reciprocal ST-segment depression in aVR, not in aVL Elevation seldom >5 mm PR-segment depression
Hyperkalemia	Other features of hyperkalemia present: • widened QRS and tall, peaked, tented T-waves • low-amplitude or absent P-waves • ST-segment usually downsloping
Brugada syndrome	rSR' in V1 and V2 ST-segment elevation in V1 and V2, typically downsloping
Pulmonary embolism	Changes simulating myocardial infarction seen often in both inferior and anteroseptal leads
Cardioversion	Striking ST-segment elevation, often >10 mm, but lasting only 1–2 minutes immediately after direct-current shock
Prinzmetal's angina	Same as ST-segment elevation in infarction, but transient
Acute myocardial infarction	ST-segment with a plateau or shoulder or upsloping Reciprocal behavior between aVL and III

Reproduced with permission from Wang *et al.* [13].

sions are intermediate risk. The magnitude of ST changes as well as the number leads involved are also important. As valuable as the electrocardiogram is, there are special circumstances where it is difficult or impossible to interpret. The electrocardiogram may be negative or nondiagnostic in more than one-half of non-ST-elevation ACS patients (*see* Figure 3.3) [15].

It is still possible to interpret ST changes in patients with right bundle branch block; however, this is much more challenging in patients with a left bundle branch block. Unfortunately, patients who present with a left bundle branch block have worse outcomes when compared with those who have interpretable electrocardiograms. While a left bundle branch block is usually the result of an extensive myocardial infarction, these patients are slow to be diagnosed and therefore experience delays in receiving reperfusion therapy. Other than having a high index of suspicion in patients with a left bundle branch block, there are electrocardiographic criteria that can aid in making the diagnosis of acute myocardial infarction more likely (*see* Figure 3.4) [16]. These consist of:

- 1 mm or more of ST-depression in V1 to V3;
- 5 mm of ST-elevation discordant to the QRS complex;
- 1 mm of ST-elevation concordant to the QRS complex.

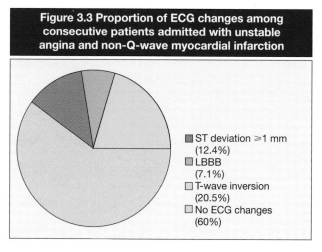

Figure 3.3 Proportion of ECG changes among consecutive patients admitted with unstable angina and non-Q-wave myocardial infarction

- ST deviation ≥1 mm (12.4%)
- LBBB (7.1%)
- T-wave inversion (20.5%)
- No ECG changes (60%)

ECG, electrocardiogram; LBBB, left bundle branch block; MI, myocardial infarction. Reproduced with permission from Cannon *et al*. [15].

Figure 3.4 Odds ratios and scoring system for predicting myocardial infarction among patients with left bundle branch block

Criterion	Odds ratio (95% CI)	Score
ST-segment elevation ≥1 mm and concordant with QRS complex	25.2 (11.6–54.7)	5
ST-segment depression ≥1 mm in lead V1, V2, or V3	6.0 (1.9–19.3)	3
ST-segment elevation ≥5 mm and discordant with QRS complex	4.3 (1.8–10.6)	2

CI, confidence interval. Reproduced with permission from Sgarbossa et al. [16].

Patients with paced rhythms are another group that makes diagnosis of myocardial infarction difficult. In patients who are not pacemaker dependent, the lower rate of the pacemaker can be reset below the patient's native sinus rhythm to allow for interpretation of native ST-segments. While this may help some patients, many will have repolarization abnormalities after reverting to a native sinus rhythm, which still make ST-segments difficult to interpret. Patients with lateral myocardial infarction due to circumflex artery occlusion also deserve special mention since this area can be electrocardiographically silent.

Summary

The diagnosis of ACS patients is critically important in order to improve cardiac outcomes, including patient survival. The art of medicine and the science of diagnostic studies combine to formulate an accurate diagnosis and assess patient risk. Novel biomarkers are under study that may allow even earlier detection of lower thresholds of myonecrosis, while electrocardiograms with greater than 12 leads are also under investigation for the diagnosis of ACS with even more precision.

References

1.   Bavry AA, Kumbhani DJ, Rassi AN, et al. Benefit of early invasive therapy in acute coronary syndromes: a meta-analysis of contemporary randomized clinical trials. J Am Coll Cardiol 2006; 48:1319–1325.

2.   Pope JH, Aufderheide TP, Ruthazer R, et al. Missed diagnoses of acute cardiac ischemia in the emergency department. N Engl J Med 2000; 342:1163–1170.

3.   Lewis WR, Amsterdam EA, Turnipseed S, *et al*. Immediate exercise testing of low risk patients with known coronary artery disease presenting to the emergency department with chest pain. *J Am Coll Cardiol* 1999; **33**:1843–1847.

4.   Milner KA, Vaccarino V, Arnold AL, *et al*. Gender and age differences in chief complaints of acute myocardial infarction (Worcester Heart Attack Study). *Am J Cardiol* 2004; **93**:606–608.

5.   Bugiardini R, Bairey Merz CN. Angina with "normal" coronary arteries: a changing philosophy. *JAMA* 2005; **293**:477–484.

6.   Braunwald E. Unstable angina. A classification. *Circulation* 1989; **80**:410–414.

7.   Lee TH, Cook EF, Weisberg M, *et al*. Acute chest pain in the emergency room. Identification and examination of low-risk patients. *Arch Intern Med* 1985; **145**:65–69.

8.   Henrikson CA, Howell EE, Bush DE, *et al*. Chest pain relief by nitroglycerin does not predict active coronary artery disease. *Ann Intern Med* 2003; **139**:979–986.

9.   Zimmerman J, Fromm R, Meyer D, *et al*. Diagnostic marker cooperative study for the diagnosis of myocardial infarction. *Circulation* 1999; **99**:1671–1677.

10.   Rajagopal V, Bhatt DL. Acute coronary syndrome statistics: what you don't see can hurt you. *Am Heart J* 2005; **149**:955–956.

11.   Aviles RJ, Askari AT, Lindahl B, *et al*. Troponin T levels in patients with acute coronary syndromes, with or without renal dysfunction. *N Engl J Med* 2002; **346**:2047–2052.

12.   Galla JG, Mahaffey KW, Sapp SK, *et al*. Elevated creatine kinase-MB with normal creatine kinase predicts worse outcomes in patients with acute coronary syndromes: results from 4 large clinical trials. *Am Heart J* 2006; **151**:16–24.

13.   Wang K, Asinger RW, Marriott HJ. ST-segment elevation in conditions other than acute myocardial infarction. *N Engl J Med* 2003; **349**:2128–2135.

14.   Savonitto S, Ardissino D, Granger CB, *et al*. Prognostic value of the admission electrocardiogram in acute coronary syndromes. *JAMA* 1999; **281**:707–713.

15.   Cannon CP, McCabe CH, Stone PH, *et al*. The electrocardiogram predicts one-year outcome of patients with unstable angina and non-Q wave myocardial infarction: results of the TIMI III Registry ECG Ancillary Study. Thrombolysis in Myocardial Ischemia. *J Am Coll Cardiol* 1997; **30**:133–140.

16.   Sgarbossa EB, Pinski SL, Barbagelata A, *et al*. Electrocardiographic diagnosis of evolving acute myocardial infarction in the presence of left bundle-branch block. GUSTO-1 (Global Utilization of Streptokinase and Tissue Plasminogen Activator for Occluded Coronary Arteries) Investigators. *N Engl J Med* 1996; **334**:481–487.

Chapter 4

Risk stratification

Patients who present with ACS should continually undergo risk stratification throughout their hospitalization. Risk stratification is synonymous with prognosis determination: patients who have the highest risk will also have the poorest prognosis. This process begins at the moment of initial medical contact, proceeds throughout hospitalization and continues thereafter. The process of risk stratification channels intensive medical care to those who are most in need, while reserving more conservative therapy for patients at lower risk. This process is essential since intensive medical care can produce its own side effects. Such side effects may be acceptable in patients at highest risk, although in lower risk populations they will become unattractive.

Risk stratification for ST-elevation myocardial infarction is mainly used to predict prognosis, unlike non-ST-elevation ACS, where risk stratification also helps to guide therapy. For such patients, the decision focuses on deciding if and when invasive therapy through left-heart catheterization and possible revascularization should take place. Patients at low risk will be able to forego invasive therapy and undergo more traditional means of risk stratification, such as stress testing, while the lowest risk patients can usually be managed with early hospital discharge. Risk stratification also identifies which patients will need the most aggressive adjuvant therapies such as anti-platelet and anti-thrombotic medications. ACS are different from stable coronary artery disease in that patients with ACS are at persistently increased risk for recurrent events. Continued risk stratification after stabilization of an ACS therefore works to limit these recurrent events through control of cardiovascular risk factors. The following sections will discuss risk stratification of ACS and focus on popular risk stratification models. Various models are specific to non-ST-elevation ACS, while others apply to ST-elevation myocardial infarction.

Variables, such as electrocardiographic changes and elevated biomarkers, are important, although when used independently they fail to fully predict a patient's risk. For electrocardiographic changes, there is a spectrum of risk where small T-wave inversions predict the lowest risk, and ST-elevation along with areas of depression predict higher risk [1]. Similarly for biomarkers, there is also a spectrum of risk that rises with increasing levels of cardiac biomarkers [2]. Since only looking at one variable may not fully predict

A.A. Bavry, D.L. Bhatt (eds.), Acute Coronary Syndromes in Clinical Practice
DOI 10.1007/978-1-84800-358-3_4, © Springer-Verlag London Limited 2009

prognosis, attempts have been made to construct accurate and easy-to-use risk models that incorporate multiple variables.

Non-ST-elevation ACS risk models

The TIMI (Thrombolysis in Myocardial Infarction) risk score is one of the more recognizable scoring systems to assess patient risk [3]. This model was incorporated from the TIMI 11B and ESSENCE (Efficacy and Safety of Subcutaneous Enoxaparin in Unstable Angina and Non-Q-Wave MI) trials and is therefore applicable to patients with unstable angina and non-ST-elevation myocardial infarction. The TIMI risk score is also useful in predicting which ACS patients will have a more favorable response to early invasive therapy when compared to medical management. The TACTICS (Treat Angina with Aggrastat and Determine the Cost of Therapy with an Invasive or Conservative Strategy)-TIMI 18 trial identified patients with an intermediate or high TIMI risk score who benefited from early invasive therapy, although the lowest risk patients appeared to do equally well on either approach [4].

The TIMI risk score incorporates seven variables (1 point for each variable) that independently predict a composite of death, myocardial infarction, or urgent revascularization at 14 days. The seven variables used in the scoring system are readily available and therefore allow for quick risk assessment (*see* Figure 4.1). They include the following characteristics [5]:

- age 65 years or greater;
- the presence of three or more traditional risk factors for coronary disease;
- previously documented coronary artery disease (i.e., ≥50% stenosis);
- the use of aspirin within the last 7 days;
- two or more angina episodes in the previous 24 hours;
- electrocardiographic changes indicative of ischemia;
- elevated cardiac biomarkers.

Patients with the highest risk (seven out of seven variables) have a composite event rate of 40%, compared with an event rate of 4.7% for the lowest risk

Figure 4.1 Variables used to construct the GRACE, TIMI and PURSUIT risk scores

	Risk score
GRACE (0–258)	
Age (years)	
<40	0
40–49	18
50–59	36
60–69	55
70–79	73
≥80	91
Heart rate (bpm)	
<70	0
70–89	7
90–109	13
110–149	23
150–199	36
≥200	46
Systolic blood pressure (mmHg)	
<80	63
80–99	58
100–119	47
120–139	37
140–159	26
160–199	11
≥200	0
Creatinine (mg/dL)	
0–0.39	2
0.4–0.79	5
0.8–1.19	8
1.2–1.59	11
1.6–1.99	14
2–3.99	23
≥4	31

CCS, Canadian Cardiovascular Society Functional Classification of Angina; GRACE, Global Registry of Acute Coronary Events; MI, myocardial infarction; PURSUIT, Platelet glycoprotein IIb/IIIa in Unstable angina: Receptor Suppression Using Integrilin Therapy; TIMI, Thrombolysis in Myocardial Infarction; UA, unstable angina. Reproduced with permission from de Araujo Goncalves [5]. *Continued overleaf*.

Figure 4.1 *Continued*. Variables used to construct the GRACE, TIMI and PURSUIT risk scores

	Risk score
Killip class	
Class I	0
Class II	21
Class III	43
Class IV	64
Cardiac arrest at admission	43
Elevated cardiac markers	64
ST-segment deviation	30
TIMI (0–7)	
Age ≥65 years	1
≥3 risk factors for coronary artery disease	1
Use of aspirin (last 7 days)	1
Known coronary artery disease (stenosis ≥50%)	1
>1 episode of rest angina in <24 hours	1
ST-segment deviation	1
Elevated cardiac markers	1
PURSUIT (0–18)	
Age [separate points for enrollment diagnosis, UA (MI)]	
50–59	8 (11)
60–69	9 (12)
70–79	11 (13)
≥80	12 (14)
Sex	
Male	1
Female	0
Worst CCS class in previous 6 weeks	
No angina or CCS I/II	0
CCS III/IV	2
Signs of heart failure	2
ST-depression on presenting electrocardiogram	1

patients (*see* Figure 4.2). The incidence of individual outcomes is similarly increased with increased risk scores (*see* Figure 4.3). The TIMI risk score has been validated to be accurate and it is easy to use; however, several important

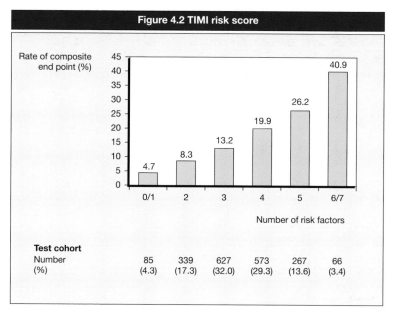

Figure 4.2 TIMI risk score

MI, myocardial infarction; TIMI, Thrombolysis In Myocardial Infarction. Reproduced with permission from Antman *et al.* [3].

caveats associated with its use should be highlighted. Patients who present with elevated biomarkers (i.e., non-ST-elevation myocardial infarction) without any other TIMI risk score variables should still receive early invasive therapy, even though this model would have predicted low risk for future events. Accordingly, for this model to effectively predict which patients will benefit from invasive therapy, it is likely best reserved for individuals with unstable angina and those with chest pain of unclear etiology. Among these individuals, the TIMI risk score can provide excellent prognostic information that can be used to determine the degree of anti-platelet and anti-thrombin therapy as well as the need for early invasive therapy. Another concern is that this model does not incorporate heart or renal failure into the scoring system, which are known to be poor prognosticators.

The PURSUIT (Platelet glycoprotein IIb/IIIa in Unstable angina: Receptor Suppression Using Integrilin [eptifibatide] Therapy) trial studied 9461

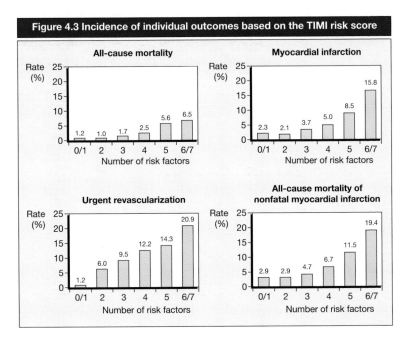

Figure 4.3 Incidence of individual outcomes based on the TIMI risk score

TIMI, Thrombolysis In Myocardial Infarction. Reproduced with permission from Antman *et al.* [3].

patients with non-ST-elevation ACS. This trial was used to construct the PURSUIT risk score that predicts death as well as death or myocardial infarction at 30 days (*see* Figure 4.4) [6]. A strength of the PURSUIT scoring system is that unlike the TIMI risk score, heart failure is included as an important prognosticator (*see* Figure 4.1) [5].

The GRACE (Global Registry of Acute Coronary Events) registry enrolled 11,389 patients across the spectrum of ACS, including ST-elevation myocardial infarction. This registry was used to construct the GRACE risk score, which predicts in-hospital adverse cardiac events through the use of eight variables (*see* Figure 4.5) [7]. Similar to the TIMI and PURSUIT risk models, GRACE incorporates advanced age and signs of heart failure, but it is unique in that it additionally adds renal insufficiency as an important prognosticator of risk (*see* Figure 4.1) [5]. This model is somewhat more cumbersome than the TIMI risk model in that there is a wide range of possible points for each variable.

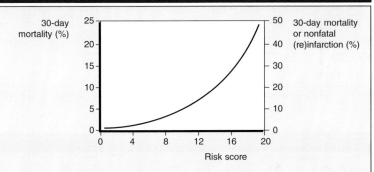

Figure 4.4 PURSUIT risk score for predicting short-term adverse outcomes among patients with non-ST-elevation ACS

	Score	
	Mortality only	Mortality or infarction
Age		
50	0	8 (11)
60	2(3)	9 (12)
70	4 (6)	11 (13)
80	6 (9)	12 (14)
Gender		
Female	0	0
Male	1	1
Worst CCS-class in previous 6 weeks		
No angina; I or II	0	0
III or IV	2	2
Heart rate (bpm)		
80	0	0
100	1 (2)	0
120	2 (5)	0
Systolic blood pressure (mmHg)		
No	0	0
Yes	3	1
Signs of heart failure (rales)		
No	0	0
Yes	3	2
ST depression on presenting ECG		
No	0	0
Yes	3	1

bpm, beats per minute; CCS, Canadian Cardiovascular Society; ECG, electrocardiogram; PURSUIT, Platelet glycoprotein IIb/IIIa in Unstable angina: Receptor Suppression Using Integrilin Therapy. Reproduced with permission from Boersma *et al.* [6].

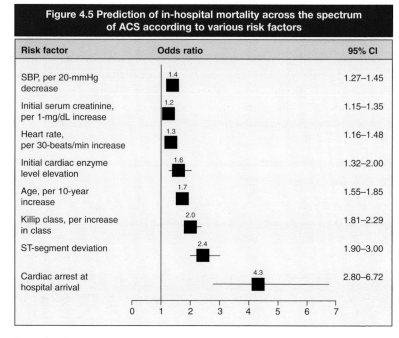

Figure 4.5 Prediction of in-hospital mortality across the spectrum of ACS according to various risk factors

Risk factor	Odds ratio	95% CI
SBP, per 20-mmHg decrease	1.4	1.27–1.45
Initial serum creatinine, per 1-mg/dL increase	1.2	1.15–1.35
Heart rate, per 30-beats/min increase	1.3	1.16–1.48
Initial cardiac enzyme level elevation	1.6	1.32–2.00
Age, per 10-year increase	1.7	1.55–1.85
Killip class, per increase in class	2.0	1.81–2.29
ST-segment deviation	2.4	1.90–3.00
Cardiac arrest at hospital arrival	4.3	2.80–6.72

CI, confidence interval; SBP, systolic blood pressure. Reproduced with permission from Granger *et al.* [7].

The TIMI, PURSUIT and GRACE models have been compared to each other for their ability to predict short-term as well as long-term adverse events [5]. All three models were found to have good discriminatory ability in the short term, which is not surprising since this is the time period for which they were designed to predict. There were differences, however, in the discriminative ability of these models to predict long-term events. The GRACE model was found to most accurately predict long-term events, which may be due to the inclusion of renal insufficiency as an important prognosticator. Similar to the analysis from the TACTICS-TIMI 18 trial, patients with the highest risk were found to derive the most benefit from invasive therapy.

In the CRUSADE (Can Rapid Risk Stratification of Unstable Angina Patients Suppress Adverse Outcomes With Early Implementation of the ACC/AHA

Guidelines) registry, fewer than 50% of the patients with an ACS underwent invasive therapy within 48 hours of hospital presentation. Patients who underwent early invasive therapy were shown to have improved survival (*see* Figure 4.6) [8,9]. Unfortunately, research has shown that patients with the poorest prognosis are less likely to receive invasive therapy even though they are most in need of it (*see* Figure 4.7) [10]. For example among non-ST-elevation ACS, 40% of the lowest risk patients received percutaneous coronary intervention in contrast to 25% of the highest risk patients.

ST-elevation risk models

As mentioned previously, the GRACE risk score can be applied across the spectrum of ACS; however, there are additional models designed specifically for ST-elevation myocardial infarction. One of the earliest models of risk stratification within the modern era of reperfusion therapy for acute myocardial

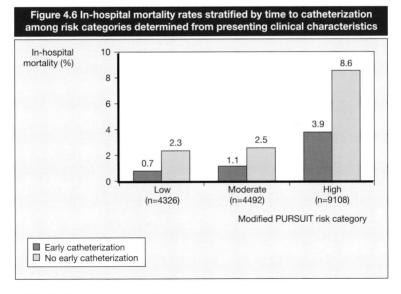

Figure 4.6 In-hospital mortality rates stratified by time to catheterization among risk categories determined from presenting clinical characteristics

PURSUIT, Platelet glycoprotein IIb/IIIa in Unstable angina: Receptor Suppression Using Integrilin Therapy. Reproduced with permission from Bhatt *et al*. [9].

Figure 4.7 The management of patients with ACS based on their GRACE risk score

	Unstable angina/NSTEMI				STEMI			
	Low risk	Medium risk	High risk	p-value	Low risk	Medium risk	High risk	p-value
Number	3944	5440	5704		4119	2623	2359	
Cardiac catheterization	2836 (72%)	3689 (68%)	2894 (51%)	<0.001	3236 (79%)	1937 (74%)	1342 (57%)	<0.001
PCI	1554 (40%)	1907 (35%)	1426 (25%)	<0.001	2466 (60%)	1421 (54%)	959 (41%)	0.98
CABG	298 (7.6%)	425 (7.9%)	361 (6.4%)	0.006	162 (4.0%)	108 (4.2%)	86 (3.7%)	0.67
Fibrinolytics	113 (2.9%)	103 (1.9%)	108 (1.9%)	0.001	1538 (38%)	828 (32%)	445 (19%)	<0.001
Exercise tolerance test	977 (25%)	1205 (23%)	915 (16%)	<0.001	807 (20%)	414 (16%)	238 (10%)	<0.001
Echocardiography	2096 (54%)	2784 (52%)	3250 (58%)	<0.001	2985 (74%)	1982 (76%)	1815 (78%)	0.002
In-hospital drugs								
Aspirin	3705 (94%)	5080 (93%)	5136 (90%)	<0.001	3948 (96%)	2490 (95%)	2147 (91%)	<0.001
Thienopyridine	2009 (52%)	2627 (49%)	2292 (41%)	<0.001	2543 (62%)	1485 (57%)	1013 (44%)	<0.001
UFH	1956 (50%)	2496 (47%)	2627 (47%)	0.001	2552 (63%)	1527 (59%)	1280 (55%)	<0.001
LMWH	2263 (58%)	3145 (58%)	3160 (56%)	0.016	2052 (50%)	1447 (56%)	1251 (54%)	<0.001
GPIIb/IIIa inhibitor	1008 (26%)	1197 (22%)	1002 (18%)	<0.001	1669 (41%)	914 (35%)	659 (28%)	0.099
ACE inhibitor	2157 (55%)	2911 (54%)	3234 (57%)	0.004	2796 (68%)	1861 (71%)	1589 (68%)	0.01
Beta-blocker	3352 (85%)	4533 (84%)	4251 (75%)	<0.001	3706 (90%)	2217 (85%)	1615 (69%)	<0.001
Calcium antagonist	1120 (29%)	1745 (32%)	1936 (34%)	<0.001	578 (14%)	490 (19%)	425 (18%)	<0.001

ACE, angiotensin-converting enzyme; CABG, coronary artery bypass grafting; GP, glycoprotein; GRACE, GLobal Registry of Acute Coronary Events; LMWH, low-molecular-weight heparin; MI, myocardial infarction; NSTEMI, non-ST-segment elevation myocardial infarction; PCI, percutaneous coronary intervention; STEMI, ST segment elevation myocardial infarction; UFH, unfractionated heparin. Reproduced with permission from Fox et al. [10].

infarction came from the GUSTO-1 (Global Utilization of Streptokinase and Tissue Plasminogen Activator for Occluded Coronary Arteries) trial [11]. This landmark trial examined the effect of various thrombolytic regimens on patients with ST-elevation myocardial infarction. This model showed that five variables can predict 90% of patient mortality at 30 days. These variables include:

- advanced age (i.e., greater than 75 years);
- Killip class III or IV heart failure;
- low systolic blood pressure;
- elevated heart rate;
- anterior myocardial infarction.

Of these variables, age is the strongest predictor of mortality. Patients younger than 45 years of age have a mortality of 1.1%, compared with 20.5% for patients older than 75 years. The theme of advanced age and hemodynamic instability as strong predictors of mortality and adverse events is also seen in more recent risk models.

The TIMI risk score for ST-elevation myocardial infarction accurately predicts 30-day mortality through the use of eight variables. Mortality among the lowest risk patients is less than 1%, although it is as high as 36% among the highest risk patients. Just as in the non-ST-elevation risk models, age and signs of heart failure predict most of the risk, although the location of the event (i.e., anterior myocardial infarction), low body weight (i.e., <67 kg), and a delay in time until treatment (i.e., >4 hours) are also important (see Figure 4.8) [12].

Given the emergent nature of ST-elevation myocardial infarction, a complete risk assessment that requires the assessment of multiple variables may be somewhat problematic. A pared down risk score with only three variables has recently been proposed [13], although this may not be ideal in all circumstances [14]. The three variables are: advanced age (i.e., greater than 80 years), presence of cardiogenic shock, and presence of heart failure.

Patients with ACS are not only at risk for short-term events, but they are also at increased risk for future events. The index hospitalization is an excellent opportunity to emphasize risk-factor modification, healthy diet, and exercise, which together can act to reduce these late events. Pharmacologically, it is now appreciated that the initiation of statin therapy

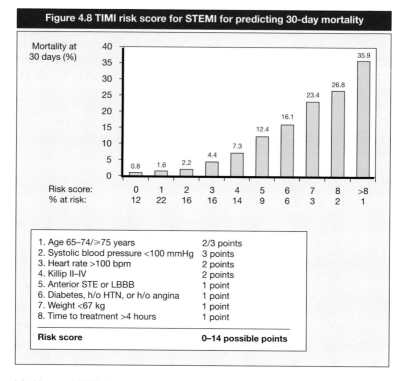

Figure 4.8 TIMI risk score for STEMI for predicting 30-day mortality

h/o, history of; HTN, hypertension; LBBB, left bundle branch block; STE, ST-elevation; STEMI, ST-elevation myocardial infarction; TIMI, Thrombolysis In Myocardial Infarction. Reproduced with permission from Morrow *et al.* [12].

during hospitalization and its continued use is associated with improved survival as well as reduced episodes of unstable angina and need for revascularization [15].

Summary

There is no perfect risk score for ACS since there is a balance between being comprehensive and completely predictive of risk versus being quick and simple, which may be accurate, although lack in discriminative ability. For non-ST-elevation ACS, the TIMI, PURSUIT and GRACE models all work well in predicting risk in the short term. The TIMI risk score is the easiest to use and can be committed to memory or referenced with a pocket card, although this model does not incorporate important variables such as heart failure and renal insufficiency. For finer estimation of risk, the GRACE score performs very well, especially for the prediction of long-term events. For ST-elevation myocardial infarction, both the TIMI and GUSTO risk scores are excellent, although if time does not allow for complete risk assessment, age and signs of cardiogenic shock or heart failure provide a good snapshot of risk.

References

1.   Savonitto S, Ardissino D, Granger CB, *et al*. Prognostic value of the admission electrocardio-gram in acute coronary syndromes. *JAMA* 1999; **281**:707–713.

2.   Antman EM, Tanasijevic MJ, Thompson B, *et al*. Cardiac-specific troponin I levels to predict the risk of mortality in patients with acute coronary syndromes. *N Engl J Med* 1996; **335**:1342–1349.

3.   Antman EM, Cohen M, Bernink PJ, *et al*. The TIMI risk score for unstable angina/non-ST elevation MI: A method for prognostication and therapeutic decision making. *JAMA* 2000; **284**:835–842.

4.   Cannon CP, Weintraub WS, Demopoulos LA, *et al*. Comparison of early invasive and con-servative strategies in patients with unstable coronary syndromes treated with the glycoprotein IIb/IIIa inhibitor tirofiban. *N Engl J Med* 2001; **344**:1879–1887.

5.   de Araujo Goncalves P, Ferreira J, Aguiar C, *et al*. TIMI, PURSUIT, and GRACE risk scores: sustained prognostic value and interaction with revascularization in NSTE-ACS. *Eur Heart J* 2005; **26**:865–872.

6.   Boersma E, Pieper KS, Steyerberg EW, *et al*. Predictors of outcome in patients with acute coronary syndromes without persistent ST-segment elevation. Results from an international trial of 9461 patients. The PURSUIT Investigators. *Circulation* 2000; **101**:2557–2567.

7.   Granger CB, Goldberg RJ, Dabbous O, *et al*. Predictors of hospital mortality in the global registry of acute coronary events. *Arch Intern Med* 2003; **163**:2345–2353.

8.   Bhatt DL. To cath or not to cath: that is no longer the question. *JAMA* 2005; **293**:2935–2937.

9.   Bhatt DL, Roe MT, Peterson ED, *et al*. Utilization of early invasive management strategies for high-risk patients with non-ST-segment elevation acute coronary syndromes: results from the CRUSADE Quality Improvement Initiative. *JAMA* 2004; **292**:2096–2104.

10.   Fox KA, Anderson FA, Jr., Dabbous OH, *et al*. Intervention in acute coronary syndromes: do patients undergo intervention on the basis of their risk characteristics? The Global Registry of Acute Coronary Events (GRACE). *Heart* 2007; **93**:177–182.

11.   Lee KL, Woodlief LH, Topol EJ, *et al*. Predictors of 30-day mortality in the era of reperfusion for acute myocardial infarction. Results from an international trial of 41,021 patients. GUSTO-I Investigators. *Circulation* 1995; **91**:1659–1668.

12.   Morrow DA, Antman EM, Charlesworth A, *et al*. TIMI risk score for ST-elevation myocardial infarction: A convenient, bedside, clinical score for risk assessment at presentation: An intravenous nPA for treatment of infarcting myocardium early II trial substudy. *Circulation* 2000; **102**:2031–2037.

13.   Negassa A, Monrad ES, Bang JY, *et al*. Tree-structured risk stratification of in-hospital mortality following percutaneous coronary intervention for acute myocardial infarction. *Am Heart J* 2007; **154**:322–329.

14.   Bavry AA, Bhatt DL. Designing the ideal risk model for acute coronary syndromes – is simple better than complex? *Am Heart J* 2007; **154**:206–207.

15.   Bavry AA, Mood GR, Kumbhani DJ, *et al*. Long-term benefit of statin therapy initiated during hospitalization for an acute coronary syndrome: a systematic review of randomized trials. *Am J Cardiovasc Drugs* 2007; **7**:135–141.

Chapter 5

Anti-platelet therapies

Anti-platelet drugs are one of the fundamental therapies for improving cardiovascular outcomes among ACS patients. Medications are used adjunctively along with mechanical or chemical reperfusion. Patients who are not candidates for revascularization may only receive medical treatment for their ACS. Cardiovascular drugs are given with the expectation that they will produce a significant beneficial effect. For some drugs in certain groups of patients, the goal is to improve survival and reduce infarct size, while for other drugs the goal is the amelioration of ischemic symptoms. Drugs, like aspirin, are widely used across the spectrum of ACS, although other agents like fibrinolytics are only used in ST-elevation myocardial infarction. It is also important to understand that each drug comes with the potential for side effects. Accordingly, the risk–benefit profile for each cardiovascular drug should be known, and the side effects minimized where possible. For some patients, the risk of a drug will outweigh its expected benefit, and should therefore not be used. This chapter will review the important anti-platelet cardiovascular drugs across the spectrum of ACS and emphasize the benefits and side effects of each agent.

Aspirin

Aspirin is the unequivocal cornerstone of cardiovascular drugs. This agent acts by irreversibly blocking platelet cyclooxygenase, which subsequently blocks thromboxane A_2 production. It is also one of the most widely studied agents. The Anti-Platelet Trialists' Collaboration studied the use of aspirin for the secondary prevention of cardiovascular events in over 100,000 patients with various forms of vascular disease [1]. Among acute myocardial infarction patients, the use of aspirin results in a 33% reduction in vascular events [1] and a 25% reduction in vascular death [2] when compared to placebo. This analysis also found that aspirin benefits patients who had remote myocardial infarction, as well as patients with stable or unstable angina, peripheral arterial disease, or history of transient ischemic attack or stroke, although low-risk patients did not clearly benefit [1]. Other findings from this analysis were that low-dose aspirin (i.e., 75–150 mg/day) is effective [1], which supports the current recommendation of low-dose aspirin for chronic therapy.

A.A. Bavry, D.L. Bhatt (eds.), Acute Coronary Syndromes in Clinical Practice   37
DOI 10.1007/978-1-84800-358-3_5, © Springer-Verlag London Limited 2009

Aspirin can result in serious bleeding in a significant proportion of patients. An important substudy from the CURE (Clopidogrel in Unstable angina to prevent Recurrent Events) trial studied the effect of various doses of aspirin [3]. This study found that major bleeding was associated with increased doses of chronic aspirin (i.e., greater than 200 mg versus less than 100 mg) whether aspirin was used alone or in combination with clopidogrel (*see* Figure 5.1). Additionally, there was some suggestion of potentially diminished efficacy with increasing doses of chronic aspirin.

Aspirin recommendation

Patients across the spectrum of ACS, from unstable angina to ST-elevation myocardial infarction, should receive 162–325 mg/day of aspirin upon hospital presentation [4,5]. Low-dose (i.e., 75–162 mg/day) should be used long term to minimize bleeding complications. New guidelines recommend aspirin 162–325 mg/day among patients who receive a coronary stent (3 months for a sirolimus stent and 6 months for a paclitaxel stent), then decrease to 75–162 mg/day [4,6]. The use of ibuprofen is discouraged due to an interaction with aspirin; however, if this medicine is used it should be given at least 8 hours before or 30 minutes after the administration of aspirin [4].

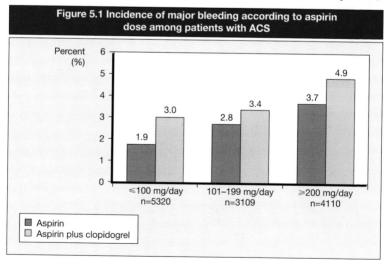

Figure 5.1 Incidence of major bleeding according to aspirin dose among patients with ACS

Reproduced with permission from Peters *et al.* [3].

Clopidogrel

Clopidogrel is a relatively new cardiovascular agent that acts by irreversibly blocking the platelet adenosine diphosphate (ADP) receptor, thus preventing platelet aggregation. The CAPRIE (Clopidogrel vs Aspirin in Patients at Risk of Ischemic Events) trial documented the superiority of clopidogrel compared with aspirin in nearly 20,000 patients with vascular disease at reducing a composite of vascular death, myocardial infarction, or stroke [7,8]. Additionally, the CURE trial found that aspirin and clopidogrel (75 mg/day after a 300-mg loading dose) were superior to aspirin alone in reducing adverse cardiovascular events among patients with non-ST-elevation ACS (*see* Figure 5.2) [9]. It is important to note that the CURE trial predominately studied conservatively treated patients with ACS who were infrequently treated with glycoprotein IIb/IIIa inhibitors (<10% of study

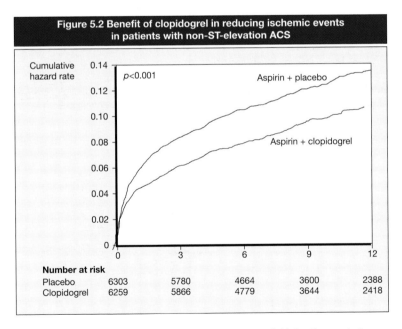

Figure 5.2 Benefit of clopidogrel in reducing ischemic events in patients with non-ST-elevation ACS

Primary outcome is a composite of death, nonfatal myocardial infarction, or stroke. Reproduced with permission from Yusuf *et al*. [9].

population) or received invasive therapy (<25% of study population); however, the patients that did undergo intervention also derived benefit from this therapy [10]. The precise role of this agent in patients with ACS who are treated aggressively with a glycoprotein IIb/IIIa inhibitor and early invasive therapy is unknown. Clopidogrel has also been shown to be beneficial in the ST-elevation myocardial infarction population [11,12]. The COMMIT (Clopidogrel and Metroprolol in Myocardial Infarction) trial studied over 45,000 patients with ST-elevation myocardial infarction, of whom half received fibrinolytic therapy (the remainder were conservatively treated) [12]. Patients randomized to clopidogrel received 75 mg/day without a loading dose for a mean of 15 days. Aspirin and clopidogrel significantly improved survival and reduced ischemic events when compared with aspirin alone. It is interesting that even though no loading dose of clopidogrel was used in this trial, the event curves began to separate early, favoring the use of clopidogrel. A meta-analysis also documented that the addition of clopidogrel to aspirin produces a small, yet significant survival advantage that is mainly restricted to the highest risk patients [13].

Clopidogrel recommendation

Clopidogrel should be used instead of aspirin in patients with ACS who have a significant allergy to aspirin [4,5]. For other patients, clopidogrel should be used in addition to aspirin early during the hospitalization [4,5]. This is especially true among patients with ACS [4], including patients with ST-elevation myocardial infarction [5]. Revascularized patients should receive 9–12 months of clopidogrel [4,5,14], or even longer for some patients (*see* Figure 5.3) [15,16], including those with a drug-eluting stent [17]. A minority of patients will require surgical revascularization, which makes the upstream use of clopidogrel (i.e., before coronary angiography) somewhat problematic, although not prohibitive, due to concerns of surgical bleeding [18]. Patients who need coronary artery bypass grafting should have clopidogrel discontinued at least 5 days before surgery is performed [4].

Prasugrel

Prasugrel is a new ADP receptor inhibitor that has been shown to be more potent and have more rapid anti-platelet effects than clopidogrel (see

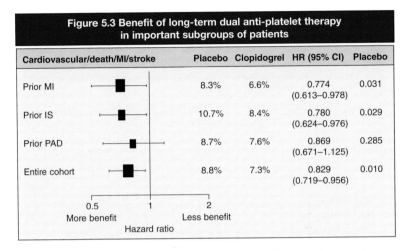

Figure 5.3 Benefit of long-term dual anti-platelet therapy in important subgroups of patients

Cardiovascular/death/MI/stroke		Placebo	Clopidogrel	HR (95% CI)	Placebo
Prior MI		8.3%	6.6%	0.774 (0.613–0.978)	0.031
Prior IS		10.7%	8.4%	0.780 (0.624–0.976)	0.029
Prior PAD		8.7%	7.6%	0.869 (0.671–1.125)	0.285
Entire cohort		8.8%	7.3%	0.829 (0.719–0.956)	0.010

0.5   1   2
More benefit   Less benefit
Hazard ratio

Mean 28 months. CI, confidence interval; HR, hazard ratio; IS, ischemic stroke; MI, myocardial infarction; PAD, peripheral arterial disease. Reproduced with permission from Bhatt et al. [16].

Figure 5.4) [19]. This agent was investigated in the TRITON-TIMI 38 (TRial to assess Improvement in Thera peutic Outcomes by optimizing platelet InhibitioN with prasugrel Thrombolysis In Myocardial Infarction 38) trial [20]. This trial randomized 13,608 moderate- to high-risk patients with ACS who underwent percutaneous coronary intervention to prasugrel or clopidogrel. Prasugrel resulted in reduced myocardial infarction, urgent target vessel revascularization, and stent thrombosis when compared to clopidogrel (see Figure 5.5) [20]. This efficacy was partially offset by increased major and life-threatening bleeding. The investigators identified three variables that produced increased bleeding with prasugrel:

- age >75 years;
- weight >60 kg;
- a history of transient ischemic attack or cerebrovascular accident.

Among patients without any of these variables, there was increased efficacy without additional major bleeding with prasugrel. Therefore, a patient's ischemic and bleeding risks will need to be assessed prior to administration of prasugrel [21].

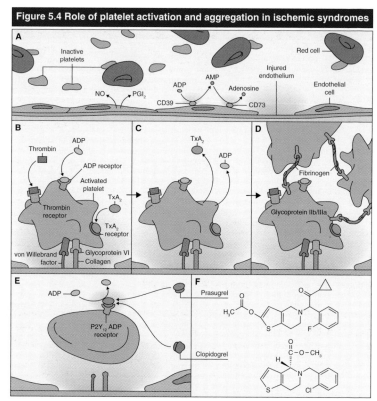

Figure 5.4 Role of platelet activation and aggregation in ischemic syndromes

(**A**) Platelets flow in the blood in their inactive state. (**B**) Several different agonists can lead to platelet activation. (**C**) The activated platelet then itself secretes prothrombotic factors. (**D**) Platelet aggregation factors. (**E**) The adenosine diphosphate (ADP) receptor plays a central role in platelet activation. (**F**) Clopidogrel and prasugrel are both thienopyridines whose active metabolites bind to the ADP receptor. AMP, adenosine monophosphate; NO, nitric oxide; PGI_2, prostacyclin; TxA_2, thromboxane A_2. Reproduced with permission from Bhatt [21].

Glycoprotein IIb/IIIa inhibitors

Glycoprotein IIb/IIIa inhibitors are agents that prevent platelet aggregation by terminally blocking platelet fibrinogen receptors. Unlike oral glycoprotein IIb/IIIa inhibitors, which have been shown to increase mortality when compared with placebo [22,23], the intravenous agents are effective in select

Figure 5.5 Major efficacy and bleeding end points in the overall TRITON-TIMI 38 cohort at 15 months			
Outcome	Incidence with prasugrel (%)	Incidence with clopidogrel (%)	Hazard ratio (95% CI)
Efficacy end points			
Cardiovascular death, myocardial infarction, or stroke	9.9	12.1	0.81 (0.73–0.90)
Myocardial infarction	7.3	9.5	0.76 (0.67–0.85)
Urgent target vessel revascularization	2.5	3.7	0.66 (0.54–0.81)
Stent thrombosis	1.1	2.4	0.48 (0.36–0.64)
Bleeding end points			
Major bleeding	2.4	1.8	1.32 (1.03–1.68)
Life-threatening bleeding	1.4	0.9	1.52 (1.08–2.13)
Fatal bleeding	0.4	0.1	4.19 (1.58–11.11)
Death, myocardial infarction, stroke, or major bleeding	12.2	13.9	0.87 (0.79–0.95)

CI, confidence interval. Adapted from Wiviott et al. [20].

patients [24]. These are now a relatively mature group of cardiovascular drugs that have been studied in numerous trials in tens of thousands of patients. Boersma and colleagues reported the use of glycoprotein IIb/IIIa inhibitors versus placebo in over 30,000 patients with ACS who were not routinely scheduled to undergo early coronary revascularization [25]. There was no difference in mortality; however, glycoprotein IIb/IIIa inhibition reduced nonfatal myocardial infarction by 17% at 5 days, and by 8% at 30 days. While there was no survival benefit in unselected patients, glycoprotein IIb/IIIa inhibitors may improve survival in conservatively treated patients with diabetes [26]. Karvouni and colleagues restricted their analysis to 20,137 patients with non-ST-elevation ACS treated with glycoprotein IIb/IIIa inhibitors versus placebo who routinely underwent percutaneous coronary intervention [27]. In this population, the adjunctive use of glycoprotein IIb/IIIa inhibitors during coronary revascularization produced a long-term survival advantage. In ST-elevation myocardial infarction, the use of abciximab compared with placebo was also associated with an early and long-term survival advantage [28]. Glycoprotein IIb/IIIa inhibitors increase major bleeding, although this can be attenuated by using lower doses of heparin and stopping heparin after percutaneous coronary intervention [27]. Hemorrhagic strokes do not appear to be increased with glycoprotein IIb/IIIa inhibition, unless combined with fibrinolytic therapy [29]; however, with the recent findings of the FINESSE trial, this practice should become infrequent [30].

Special issues with glycoprotein IIb/IIIa inhibitors

In the above analyses, the most commonly studied agents were abciximab, eptifibatide, and tirofiban. The TARGET (Do Tirofiban and ReoPro Give Similar Efficacy Trial) study documented the superiority of abciximab in reducing death, nonfatal myocardial infarction, or urgent revascularization compared with tirofiban [31]. The reduction in the composite end point was primarily driven by a reduction in nonfatal myocardial infarction.

Glycoprotein IIb/IIIa inhibitors can be given prior to cardiac catheterization (i.e., 'upstream') or at the time of coronary intervention. In fact, there is evidence that intracoronary administration of a glycoprotein IIb/IIIa inhibitor may reduce adverse cardiac events [32] compared with intravenous administration. The ACUITY (Acute Catheterization and Urgent Intervention Triage Strategy) timing trial documented a composite ischemia rate of 7.1% with upstream administration of a glycoprotein IIb/IIIa inhibitor compared with 7.9% with deferred use (p=0.13) [33]. Unfortunately, major bleeding was increased with upstream use (6.1%), compared to deferred use (4.9%; p=0.009). The importance of this finding cannot be overstated since major bleeding significantly increases short-term mortality (*see* Figure 5.6) [34]. Further study of upstream versus deferred use of eptifibatide is underway in the EARLY ACS trial.

Glycoprotein IIb/IIIa inhibitor recommendation

Glycoprotein IIb/IIIa inhibitors are best suited for patients with ACS who undergo percutaneous coronary intervention [4,5]; however, conservatively treated patients with diabetes may also derive benefit from their use [26]. Abciximab appears to be preferred to the other agents when initiated in the catheterization laboratory and should be continued for 12 hours after intervention [31]. When eptifibatide and tirofiban are used, they should be continued for 18–24 hours after intervention, although if these agents are initiated upstream, eptifibatide may be preferred as it has better data for use in percutaneous coronary intervention than tirofiban [4,5]. Glycoprotein IIb/IIIa inhibitors increase major bleeding, which is a potent predictor of short-term mortality [34]. Mechanisms to reduce major bleeding include:

Figure 5.6 The impact of major bleeding on mortality from the ACUITY trial

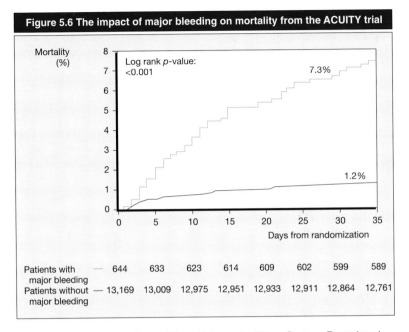

		644	633	623	614	609	602	599	589
Patients with major bleeding	—								
Patients without major bleeding	—	13,169	13,009	12,975	12,951	12,933	12,911	12,864	12,761

ACUITY, Acute Catheterization and Urgent Intervention Triage Strategy. Reproduced with permission from Manoukian [34].

proper dosing (especially for the elderly and patients with renal insufficiency) [4,5]; termination of anti-thrombin agents after revascularization [27]; and administration of glycoprotein IIb/IIIa inhibitors in the catheterization laboratory (intracoronary administration may be preferable) after arterial access has been obtained [32].

References

1. Collaborative overview of randomised trials of antiplatelet therapy – I: Prevention of death, myocardial infarction, and stroke by prolonged antiplatelet therapy in various categories of patients. Antiplatelet Trialists' Collaboration. *BMJ* 1994; **308**:81–106.

2. Randomised trial of intravenous streptokinase, oral aspirin, both, or neither among 17,187 cases of suspected acute myocardial infarction: ISIS-2. ISIS-2 (Second International Study of Infarct Survival) Collaborative Group. *Lancet* 1988; **2**:349–360.

3.   Peters RJ, Mehta SR, Fox KA, *et al.*; Clopidogrel in Unstable angina to prevent Recurrent Events (CURE) Trial Investigators. Effects of aspirin dose when used alone or in combination with clopidogrel in patients with acute coronary syndromes: observations from the Clopidogrel in Unstable angina to prevent Recurrent Events (CURE) study. *Circulation* 2003; **108**:1682–1687.

4.   Anderson JL, Adams CD, Antman EM, *et al.* ACC/AHA 2007 guidelines for the management of patients with unstable angina/non ST-elevation myocardial infarction: executive summary. A report of the American College of Cardiology/American Heart Association Task Force on practice guidelines (writing committee to revise the 2002 guidelines for the management of patients with unstable angina/non ST-elevation myocardial infarction. *Circulation* 2007; **116**:803–877.

5.   Antman EM, Anbe DT, Armstrong PW, *et al.* ACC/AHA guidelines for the management of patients with ST-elevation myocardial infarction. *Circulation* 2004; **110**:e82–e293.

6.   Smith SC Jr, Feldman TE, Hirshfeld JW Jr, *et al.* ACC/AHA/SCAI 2005 guideline update for percutaneous coronary intervention: A report of the American College of Cardiology/American Heart Association Task Force on Practice Guidelines (ACC/AHA/SCAI Writing Committee to Update the 2001 Guidelines for Percutaneous Coronary Intervention). Available at: *www.americanheart.org/presenter.jhtml?identifier=3035436*. Last accessed December 2007.

7.   A randomised, blinded, trial of clopidogrel versus aspirin in patients at risk of ischaemic events (CAPRIE). CAPRIE Steering Committee. *Lancet* 1996; **348**:1329–1339.

8.   Hirsh J, Bhatt DL. Comparative benefits of clopidogrel and aspirin in high-risk patient populations lessons from the CAPRIE and CURE Studies. *Arch Intern Med* 2004; **164**:2106–2110.

9.   Yusuf S, Zhao F, Mehta SR, *et al.* Effects of clopidogrel in addition to aspirin in patients with acute coronary syndromes without ST-segment elevation. *N Engl J Med* 2001; **345**:494–502.

10.   Mehta SR, Yusuf S, Peters RJG, *et al.*; Clopidogrel in Unstable angina to prevent Recurrent Events trial (CURE) Investigators. Effects of pretreatment with clopidogrel and aspirin followed by long-term therapy in patients undergoing percutaneous coronary intervention: the PCI-CURE study. *Lancet* 2001; **358**:527–533.

11.   Sabatine MS, Cannon CP, Gibson M, *et al.*; Clopidogrel as Adjunctive Reperfusion Therapy (CLARITY)-Thrombolysis in Myocardial Infarction (TIMI) 28 Investigators. Effect of clopidogrel pretreatment before percutaneous coronary intervention in patients with ST-elevation myocardial infarction treated with fibrinolytics: the PCI-CLARITY study. *JAMA* 2005; **294**:1224–1232.

12.   Chen ZM, Jiang LX, Chen YP, *et al.*; COMMIT (ClOpidogrel and Metoprolol in Myocardial Infarction Trial) collaborative group. Addition of clopidogrel to aspirin in 45,852 patients with acute myocardial infarction: randomised placebo-controlled trial. *Lancet* 2005; **366**:1607–1621.

13.   Helton TJ, Bavry AA, Kumbhani DJ, *et al.* Incremental effect of clopidogrel on cardiovascular outcomes in patients with vascular disease: a meta-analysis of randomized trials. *Am J Cardiovasc Drugs* 2007; **7**:289–297.

14.   Steinhubl SR, Berger PB, Mann JT, *et al.*; CREDO Investigators. Clopidogrel for the Reduction of Events During Observation. Early and sustained dual oral antiplatelet therapy following percutaneous coronary intervention: a randomized controlled trial. *JAMA* 2002; **288**:2411–2420.

15.   Bhatt DL, Fox KAA, Hacke W, *et al.*; CHARISMA Investigators. Clopidogrel and aspirin versus aspirin alone for the prevention of atherothrombotic events. *N Engl J Med* 2006; **354**:1706–1717.

16. Bhatt DL, Flather MD, Hacke W, *et al.*; CHARISMA Investigators. Patients with prior myocardial infarction, stroke, or symptomatic peripheral arterial disease in the CHARISMA Trial. *J Am Coll Cardiol* 2007; **49**:1982–1988.

17. Grines CL, Bonow RO, Casey DE Jr, *et al.* Prevention of premature discontinuation of dual antiplatelet therapy in patients with coronary artery stents: a science advisory from the American Heart Association, American College of Cardiology, Society for Cardiovascular Angiography and Interventions, American College of Surgeons, and American Dental Association, with representation from the American College of Physicians. *Circulation* 2007; **115**:813–818.

18. Bavry AA, Lincoff AM. Is clopidogrel cardiovascular medicine's double-edged sword? *Circulation* 2006; **113**:1638–1640.

19. Wiviott SD, Antman EM, Winters KJ, *et al.*; JUMBO-TIMI 26 Investigators. Randomized comparison of prasugrel (CS-747, LY640315), a novel thienopyridine P2Y12 antagonist, with clopidogrel in percutaneous coronary intervention: results of the Joint Utilization of Medications to Block Platelets Optimally (JUMBO)–TIMI 26 trial. *Circulation* 2005; **111**:3366–3373.

20. Wiviott SD, Braunwald E, McCabe CH, *et al.*; TRITON-TIMI 38 Investigators. Prasugrel versus clopidogrel in patients with acute coronary syndromes. *N Engl J Med* 2007; **357**:2001–2015.

21. Bhatt DL. Intensifying platelet inhibition – navigating between Scylla and Charybdis. *N Engl J Med* 2007; **357**:2078–2081.

22. Chew DP, Bhatt DL, Sapp S, *et al.* Increased mortality with oral platelet glycoprotein IIb/IIIa antagonists: a meta-analysis of phase III multicenter randomized trials. *Circulation* 2001; **103**:201–206.

23. Quinn MJ, Plow EF, Topol EJ. Platelet glycoprotein IIb/IIIa inhibitors: recognition of a two-edged sword? *Circulation* 2002; **106**:379–385.

24. Bhatt DL, Topol EJ. Current role of platelet glycoprotein IIb/IIIa inhibitors in acute coronary syndromes. *JAMA* 2000; **284**:1549–1558.

25. Boersma E, Harrington RA, Moliterno DJ, *et al.* Platelet glycoprotein IIb/IIIa inhibitors in acute coronary syndromes: a meta-analysis of all major randomized clinical trials. *Lancet* 2002; **359**:189–198.

26. Roffi M, Chew DP, Mukherjee D, *et al.* Platelet glycoprotein IIb/IIIa inhibitors reduce mortality in diabetic patients with non-ST-segment-elevation acute coronary syndromes. *Circulation* 2001; **104**:2767–2771.

27. Karvouni E, Katritsis DG, Ioannidis JPA. Intravenous glycoprotein IIb/IIIa receptor antagonists reduce mortality after percutaneous coronary intervention. *J Am Coll Cardiol* 2003; **41**:26–32.

28. De Luca G, Suryapranata H, Stone GW, *et al.* Abciximab as adjunctive therapy to reperfusion in acute ST-elevation myocardial infarction: a meta-analysis of randomized trials. *JAMA* 2006; **293**:1759–1765.

29. Keeley EC, Boura JA, Grines CL. Comparison of primary and facilitated percutaneous coronary interventions for ST-elevation myocardial infarction: quantitative review of randomized trials. *Lancet* 2006; **367**:579–588.

30. FINESSE: Abciximab-only- and lytic/abciximab-facilitated PCI no better than primary PCI. Available at: *www.medscape.com/viewarticle/562390*. Last accessed January 2008.

31. Topol EJ, Moliterno DJ, Herrmann HC, *et al.*; TARGET Investigators. Do Tirofiban and ReoPro Give Similar Efficacy Trial. Comparison of two platelet glycoprotein IIb/IIIa inhibitors, tirofiban and abciximab, for the prevention of ischemic events with percutaneous coronary revascularization. *N Engl J Med* 2001; **344**:1888–1894.

32. Wohrle J, Grebe OC, Nusser T, *et al.* Reduction of major adverse cardiac events with intra-coronary compared with intravenous bolus application of abciximab in patients with acute myocardial infarction or unstable angina undergoing coronary angioplasty. *Circulation* 2003; **107**:1840–1843.

33. Stone GW, Bertrand ME, Moses JW, *et al.*; ACUITY Investigators. Routine upstream initiation vs deferred selective use of glycoprotein IIb/IIIa inhibitors in acute coronary syndromes: the ACUITY timing trial. *JAMA* 2007; **297**:591–602.

34. Manoukian SV, Feit F, Mehran R, *et al.* Impact of major bleeding on 30-day mortality and clinical outcomes in patients with acute coronary syndromes: an analysis from the ACUITY trial. *J Am Coll Cardiol* 2007; **49**:1362–1368.

Chapter 6

Anti-thrombin therapy

This chapter reviews the anti-thrombin agents (also known as anti-coagulants), which include the heparins (unfractionated heparin and low-molecular heparin [i.e., enoxaparin]), direct thrombin inhibitors (i.e., biva-lirudin), and factor Xa inhibitors (i.e., fondaparinux). The interest behind the use of anti-thrombin agents stems from the fact that ACS patients who are only treated with anti-platelet agents are still at risk of significant ischemic events. The clinical trial experience with these agents crosses several decades. This span includes an early era with relatively nonaggressive anti-platelet therapies (i.e., infrequent or no aspirin, thienopyridines, glyco-protein IIb/IIIa inhibitors), or adjuvant therapies (i.e., statins). This earlier time period was also largely characterized by noninvasive therapy, which is not currently considered the standard of care for ACS patients. Accordingly, the substantial improvement in medical therapy and invasive management of patients with ACS makes interpretation of the early trial experience relatively difficult, compared with the newer cardiovascular agents. Our discussion will start with heparin, which is the oldest anti-thrombin agent in the care of ACS patients.

Unfractionated heparin

Unfractionated heparin is derived from porcine intestine and contains a wide range of sizes of polysaccharide molecules with a mean weight of approximately 15,000 Daltons. Heparin contains a pentasaccharide sequence that binds to anti-thrombin, thus indirectly inhibiting factor Xa. Unfractionated heparin is incompletely absorbed by the subcutaneous route; therefore, it must be given intravenously. Among conservatively treated ACS patients on a background of aspirin therapy, the use of unfractionated heparin significantly reduced the incidence of death or myocardial infarction compared to placebo (*see* Figure 6.1) [1]. The duration of heparin in these trials ranged from 2 to 7 days. The composite outcome was largely driven by a reduction in myocardial infarction. When the trials that reported the use of low-molec-ular-weight heparin compared to placebo were also included in this analysis, the reduction in ischemic events was even more pronounced.

A.A. Bavry, D.L. Bhatt (eds.), Acute Coronary Syndromes in Clinical Practice
DOI 10.1007/978-1-84800-358-3_6, © Springer-Verlag London Limited 2009

Figure 6.1 Benefit of UFH or LMWH compared to placebo in ACS

Study	UFH or LMWH	Control	OR	95% CI
Theroux	2/122 (1.6%)	4/121 (3.3%)	0.50	0.10–2.53
Cohen	0/37	1/32 (3.1%)	0.12	0.01–5.89
RISC	3/210 (1.4%)	7/189 (3.7%)	0.40	0.11–1.39
Cohen	4/105 (3.8%)	9/109 (8.2%)	0.46	0.15–1.41
Holdright	42/154 (27.3%)	40/131 (30.5%)	0.85	0.51–1.41
Gurfinkel (UFH)	4/70 (5.7%)	7/73 (9.6%)	0.58	0.17–1.98
Gurfinkel (LMWH)	0/68	7/73 (9.6%)	0.13	0.03–0.60
FRISC I	4/70 (5.7%)	36/757 (4.8%)	0.39	0.22–0.68
UFH vs placebo/control	55/698 (7.9%)	68/655 (10.4%)	0.67	0.45–0.99
LMWH vs placebo	13/809 (1.6%)	43/830 (5.2%)	0.34	0.20–0.58
Grand total	68/1507 (4.5%)	104/1412 (4.5%)	0.53	0.38–0.73

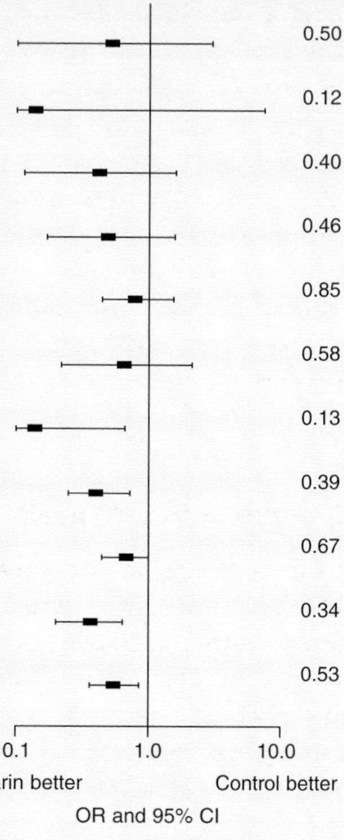

0.1   1.0   10.0

Heparin better   Control better

OR and 95% CI

CI, confidence interval; FRISC 1, fragnim during instability in coronary artery disease; LMWH, low-molecular-weight heparin; OR, odds ratio; UFH, unfractionated heparin. Reproduced with permission from Eikelboom *et al.* [1].

Unfractionated heparin is routinely given with thrombolytics and primary angioplasty for ST-elevation myocardial infarction, although the data that support this practice are relatively weak. Patients are at risk of recurrent ischemic events upon termination of heparin unless coronary revascularization has taken place [2].

Unfractionated heparin recommendation

Unfractionated heparin should be given for ACS. The dose of heparin required to achieve full anti-coagulation is 80 units/kg initial bolus (maximum of 5000 units), followed by 18 units/kg/hour infusion for an activated clotting time of at least 250 seconds [3]. However, ACS patients are often treated with adjunctive thrombolytics or glycoprotein IIb/IIIa inhibitors; therefore, the recommended weight-based heparin dose is lower. For ACS patients, the recommended heparin dose is 60 units/kg initial bolus (maximum of 4000 units), followed by 12 units/kg/hour infusion (maximum 1000 units/hour) to maintain a partial thromboplastin time of 50–75 seconds or an activated clotting time of greater than 200 seconds [4,5]. Heparin should be discontinued after stent implantation; however, angioplasty-only interventions may have a reduction in ischemic events from the use of post-procedural heparin [6].

Low-molecular-weight heparin

Low-molecular-weight heparin has a narrower range of sizes of polysaccharide molecules with a mean weight of approximately 5000 Daltons. There are pharmacological advantages of a low-molecular-weight heparin over unfractionated heparin. These include less platelet activation, predictable absorption with subcutaneous administration, and less heparin-induced thrombocytopenia. Low-molecular-weight heparin does not require monitoring except in special circumstances such as pregnancy or perhaps marked renal dysfunction, in which case anti-Xa levels can be monitored. The superiority of low-molecular-weight heparin over unfractionated heparin has been controversial, in part due to variability in trial study design. In the Eikelboom analysis, 12,171 patients were randomized to low-molecular-weight heparin versus unfractionated heparin [1]. Overall, there was no obvious difference in efficacy or safety favoring one agent over another, although various low-molecular-weight heparins were studied, which could have diminished the ability to find an association. Antman and colleagues, therefore, limited their analysis to enoxaparin versus unfractionated heparin in 7081 largely conservatively treated patients [7]. They concluded that enoxaparin resulted in a nearly 18% reduction in death or myocardial infarction at 43 days and this benefit was seen early (*see* Figure 6.2) [7]. This benefit was achieved without an increase in major bleeding.

The SYNERGY (Superior Yield of the New Strategy of Enoxaparin, Revascularization and Glycoprotein IIb/IIIa Inhibitors) study deserves special comment [8]. This was a contemporary trial in over 10,000 participants. Overall, 92% of the study participants underwent coronary angiography, 62% received clopidogrel, and 57% received a glycoprotein IIb/IIIa inhibitor. At 30 days, the incidence of death or myocardial infarction was similar between enoxaparin (14.0%) and unfractionated heparin (14.5%, $p=0.40$), although major bleeding was slightly increased by enoxaparin (*see* Figure 6.3) [8]. Part of the explanation for the increased bleeding with enoxaparin may be due to the fact that 75% of the patients received anticoagulation prior to randomization and may have crossed over from one type of therapy to another. Petersen and colleagues reported the largest meta-analysis on the topic, including nearly 22,000 patients [9]. At 30 days there was no difference in mortality, although enoxaparin resulted in a small

Figure 6.2 Enoxaparin reduces death and myocardial infarction compared to UFH

Day	UFH (%)	Enoxaparin (%)		Odds ratio (95% CI)	Reduction (%)	*p*-value
2	1.8	1.4%		0.80 (0.55–1.16)	20	0.24
8	5.3	4.2%		0.77 (0.62–0.95)	23	0.02
14	6.5	5.2%		0.79 (0.65–0.96)	21	0.02
43	8.6	7.1%		0.82 (0.69–0.97)	18	0.02

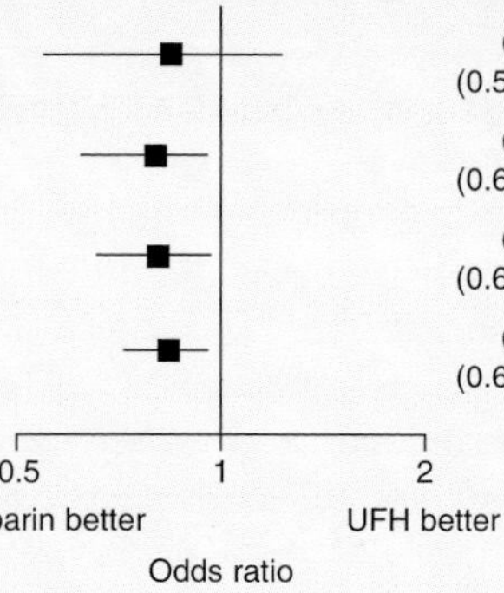

```
            0.5              1              2
       Enoxaparin better          UFH better
                    Odds ratio
```

Benefits are seen early and persist for 43 days. CI, confidence interval; UFH, unfractionated heparin. Reproduced with permission with Antman *et al.* [7].

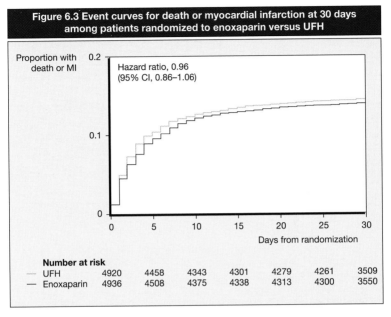

Figure 6.3 Event curves for death or myocardial infarction at 30 days among patients randomized to enoxaparin versus UFH

CI, confidence interval; UFH, unfractionated heparin. Reproduced with permission from Ferguson *et al.* [8].

(9%) reduction in myocardial infarction. There was also no difference in major bleeding at 7 days.

Two large pivotal trials in the ST-elevation myocardial population have also tested the merit of low-molecular-weight heparin. The CREATE (Clinical Trial of Reviparin and Metabolic Modulation in Acute Myocardial Infarction Treatment Evaluation) study randomized over 15,000 patients to the low-molecular-weight heparin reviparin versus placebo [10]. The study drug was administered for 7 days and 73% of the patients were treated with thrombolytic therapy. At 7 days, there was a significant reduction in death and myocardial infarction from the use of reviparin, although at the cost of increased major bleeding. There was no difference in the incidence of stroke.

The ExTRACT (Enoxaparin and Thrombolysis Reperfusion for Acute Myocardial Infarction Treatment) trial randomized over 20,000 ST-elevation myocardial infarction patients to enoxaparin versus unfractionated heparin [11]. Enoxaparin was administered for 7 days and unfractionated heparin for 2 days (consistent with the guidelines). Virtually 100% of the participants received a thrombolytic agent, of which 80% was a fibrin-specific agent. Enoxaparin did not reduce mortality, although it did decrease myocardial infarction and urgent revascularization. Major bleeding was increased with enoxaparin. Among the patients who underwent percutaneous coronary intervention, the use of enoxaparin appeared to be superior to unfractionated heparin [12]. Attention must be given to careful dosing, especially among the elderly and those with diminished renal function.

Low-molecular-weight heparin recommendation

Low-molecular-weight heparin (i.e., enoxaparin) is a reasonable alternative to unfractionated heparin for conservatively treated non-ST-elevation ACS and thrombolytic-treated ST-elevation myocardial infarction [4]. Low-molecular-weight heparin is contraindicated with a heparin allergy and requires cautious use in the elderly and patients with renal insufficiency. In the ExTRACT trial, the dose of enoxaparin was reduced in the elderly; no intravenous bolus was given and the subcutaneous dose was reduced from 1.0 mg/kg to 0.75 mg/kg twice daily [11]. For patients with an estimated creatinine clearance less than 30 cc/min, 1 mg/kg of enoxaparin was given once daily.

Direct thrombin inhibitors

These agents bind directly to thrombin (factor IIa) [13]. They may be advantageous since thrombocytopenia has only rarely been observed with their use. The ACUITY trial randomized 13,819 patients with non-ST-elevation ACS to one of the following groups [14]:

- heparin (unfractionated heparin or low-molecular-weight heparin) and a glycoprotein IIb/IIIa inhibitor;
- bivalirudin and a glycoprotein IIb/IIIa inhibitor;
- bivalirudin alone.

The regimens that included a glycoprotein IIb/IIIa inhibitor had similar efficacy and safety. The bivalirudin-alone group was noninferior to heparin plus a glycoprotein IIb/IIIa inhibitor with respect to efficacy, although it was associated with significantly less bleeding. The only subgroup where bivalirudin alone may have been inferior to heparin and a glycoprotein IIb/IIIa inhibitor was in patients not pre-treated with a thienopyridine (see Figure 6.4) [14].

Bivalirudin has also been studied in ST-elevation myocardial infarction. This agent compared favorably to heparin and a glycoprotein IIb/IIIa inhibitor by reducing cardiovascular death, myocardial infarction, and bleeding. This was partially offset by an increase in periprocedural stent thrombosis [15].

Direct thrombin inhibitor recommendation

Bivalirudin, with the option of a glycoprotein IIb/IIIa inhibitor as a bailout, is a reasonable alternative to heparin plus routine use of a glycoprotein IIb/IIIa inhibitor for non-ST-elevation ACS [4]. Bivalirudin alone may not adequately protect against ischemic events in patients not pretreated with a thienopyridine or when there may be a delay to catheterization. Bivalirudin has not been well studied in the ST-elevation myocardial infarction population, although the ongoing HORIZONS (Harmonizing Outcomes With Revascularization and Stents) trial will address this question.

Factor Xa inhibitors

Fondaparinux is the only factor Xa drug that is currently available, although others are being evaluated [16,17]. This agent is an indirect inhibitor of factor Xa and is completely absorbed after subcutaneous administration. The half-life of fondaparinux is approximately 17 hours, which makes once-daily dosing possible. The fifth OASIS (Organization to Assess Strategies in Acute Ischemic Syndromes) trial studied 20,078 patients with non-ST-elevation ACS [18]. Patients were randomized to either fondaparinux or enoxaparin. The primary outcome (death, myocardial infarction, or refractory ischemia) was similar between the two groups at 9 days. There was a 2% absolute decrease in major bleeding from the use of fondaparinux. This translated into decreased mortality at 30 days (2.9% versus 3.5%, $p=0.02$), which remained significant at 180 days (5.8% versus 6.5%, $p=0.05$). Unfortunately,

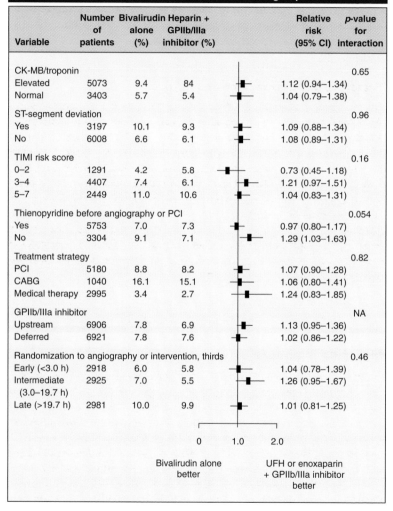

Figure 6.4 The effect of bivalirudin alone, compared to heparin and a GPIIb/IIIa inhibitor across various subgroups

Variable	Number of patients	Bivalirudin alone (%)	Heparin + GPIIb/IIIa inhibitor (%)	Relative risk (95% CI)	p-value for interaction
CK-MB/troponin					0.65
Elevated	5073	9.4	84	1.12 (0.94–1.34)	
Normal	3403	5.7	5.4	1.04 (0.79–1.38)	
ST-segment deviation					0.96
Yes	3197	10.1	9.3	1.09 (0.88–1.34)	
No	6008	6.6	6.1	1.08 (0.89–1.31)	
TIMI risk score					0.16
0–2	1291	4.2	5.8	0.73 (0.45–1.18)	
3–4	4407	7.4	6.1	1.21 (0.97–1.51)	
5–7	2449	11.0	10.6	1.04 (0.83–1.31)	
Thienopyridine before angiography or PCI					0.054
Yes	5753	7.0	7.3	0.97 (0.80–1.17)	
No	3304	9.1	7.1	1.29 (1.03–1.63)	
Treatment strategy					0.82
PCI	5180	8.8	8.2	1.07 (0.90–1.28)	
CABG	1040	16.1	15.1	1.06 (0.80–1.41)	
Medical therapy	2995	3.4	2.7	1.24 (0.83–1.85)	
GPIIb/IIIa inhibitor					NA
Upstream	6906	7.8	6.9	1.13 (0.95–1.36)	
Deferred	6921	7.8	7.6	1.02 (0.86–1.22)	
Randomization to angiography or intervention, thirds					0.46
Early (<3.0 h)	2918	6.0	5.8	1.04 (0.78–1.39)	
Intermediate (3.0–19.7 h)	2925	7.0	5.5	1.26 (0.95–1.67)	
Late (>19.7 h)	2981	10.0	9.9	1.01 (0.81–1.25)	

0   1.0   2.0

Bivalirudin alone better   UFH or enoxaparin + GPIIb/IIIa inhibitor better

CABG, coronary artery bypass graft; CK-MB, creatine kinase myocardial band isoenzyme; GP, glycoprotein; PCI, percutaneous coronary interventions; TIMI, Thrombolysis in Myocardial Infarction; UFH, unfractionated heparin. Reproduced with permission from Stone *et al.* [14].

the fondaparinux-treated group had significantly more catheter-related thrombi, which diminished enthusiasm for this agent in patients managed with an early invasive approach. Similarly, fondaparinux reduced mortality, myocardial infarction, and bleeding predominantly in thrombolytic-treated, but not primary angioplasty-treated ST-elevation myocardial infarction patients [19].

Factor Xa inhibitor recommendations

During the initial medical stabilization of patients with non-ST-elevation ACS, fondaparinux can be considered as an alternative to low-molecular-weight heparin [4]. For example, this drug could be given to patients who present on the weekend with a non-ST-elevation myocardial infarction where the decision is made to perform cardiac catheterization 1 to 2 days later. Also, if the patient is not a candidate for invasive therapy, fondaparinux would be an attractive alternative. This may also be a good agent in thrombolytic-treated ST-elevation myocardial infarction patients. Individuals who initially receive fondaparinux should be treated with heparin or bivalirudin in the catheterization laboratory if percutaneous coronary intervention is performed, although proper dosing algorithms need to be developed.

Summary

Anti-coagulation is recommended to all patients across the spectrum of ACS. Unfractionated heparin is the oldest agent and is still widely used today. It is the historical gold standard, especially during coronary intervention. Low-molecular-weight heparin may be superior to unfractionated heparin, especially in conservatively treated non-ST-elevation ACS and in thrombolytic-treated ST-elevation myocardial infarction patients. Bivalirudin is an alternative to heparin plus glycoprotein IIb/IIIa inhibition during ACS, as long as the patient has received adequate anti-platelet therapy (i.e., sufficient pretreatment with a thienopyridine). Fondaparinux should be considered given its ability to reduce major bleeding and improve survival. The caveat with fondaparinux is that coronary intervention should still take place on a background of heparin or a direct thrombin inhibitor due to the potential for catheter-related thrombi.

References

1.   Eikelboom JW, Anand SS, Malmberg K, *et al.* Unfractionated heparin and low-molecular-weight heparin in acute coronary syndrome without ST elevation: a meta-analysis. *Lancet* 2000; **355**:1936–1942.

2.   Lauer MA, Houghtaling PL, Peterson JG, *et al.* Attenuation of rebound ischemia after discontinuation of heparin therapy by glycoprotein IIb/IIIa inhibition with eptifibatide in patients with acute coronary syndromes. Observations from the Platelet IIb/IIIa in Unstable Angina: Receptor Suppression Using Integrilin Therapy (PURSUIT) Trial. *Circulation* 2001; **104**:2772–2777.

3.   Hirsh J, Raschke R. Heparin and low-molecular-weight heparin. The seventh ACCP conference on antithrombotic and thrombolytic therapy. *Chest* 2004; **126**:188S–203S.

4.   Anderson JL, Adams CD, Antman EM, *et al.* ACC/AHA 2007 guidelines for the management of patients with unstable angina/non ST-elevation myocardial infarction: executive summary. A report of the American College of Cardiology/American Heart Association Task Force on practice guidelines (writing committee to revise the 2002 guidelines for the management of patients with unstable angina/non ST-elevation myocardial infarction. *Circulation* 2007; **116**:803–877.

5.   Antman EM, Anbe DT, Armstrong PW, *et al.* ACC/AHA guidelines for the management of patients with ST-elevation myocardial infarction. *Circulation* 2004; **110**:e82–e293.

6.   Harjai KJ, Stone GW, Grines CL, *et al.* Usefulness of routine unfractionated heparin infusion following primary percutaneous coronary intervention for acute myocardial infarction in patients not receiving glycoprotein IIb/IIIa inhibitors. *Am J Cardiol* 2007; **99**:202–207.

7.   Antman, EM, Cohen M, Radley D, *et al.* Assessment of the treatment effect of enoxaparin for unstable angina/non-Q-wave myocardial infarction. TIMI 11B-ESSENCE meta-analysis. *Circulation* 1999; **100**:1602–1608.

8.   Ferguson JJ, Califf RM, Antman EM, *et al.*; SYNERGY Trial Investigators. Enoxaparin vs unfractionated heparin in high-risk patients with non-ST-segment elevation acute coronary syndromes managed with an intended early invasive strategy. Primary results of the SYNERGY randomized trial. *JAMA* 2004; **292**:45–54.

9.   Petersen JL, Mahaffey, KW, Hasselblad V, *et al.* Efficacy and bleeding complications among patients randomized to enoxaparin for unfractionated heparin for antithrombin therapy in non-ST-segment elevation acute coronary syndromes. A systematic overview. *JAMA* 2004; **292**:89–96.

10.   Yusuf S, Mehta SR, Xie C, *et al.*; CREATE Trial Group Investigators. Effects of reviparin, a low-molecular-weight heparin, on mortality, reinfarction, and strokes in patients with acute myocardial infarction presenting with ST-segment elevation. *JAMA* 2005; **293**:427–436.

11.   Antman EM, Morrow DA, McCabe CH, *et al.* Enoxaparin versus unfractionated heparin with fibrinolysis for ST-elevation myocardial infarction. *N Engl J Med* 2006; **354**:1477–1488.

12.   Gibson CM, Murphy SA, Montalescot G, *et al.* Percutaneous coronary intervention in patients receiving enoxaparin or unfractionated heparin after fibrinolytic therapy for ST-segment elevation myocardial infarction in the ExTRACT-TIMI 25 trial. *J Am Coll Cardiol* 2007; **49**:2238–2246.

13.   Gurm HS, Bhatt DL. Thrombin, an ideal target for pharmacological inhibition: a review of direct thrombin inhibitors. *Am Heart J* 2005; **149**:S43–S53.

14.   Stone GW, McLaurin BT, Cox DA, *et al.* Bivalirudin for patients with acute coronary syndromes. *N Engl J Med* 2006; **355**:2203–1226.

15.   HORIZONS AMI: Bivalirudin reduces bleeding, adverse clinical events in STEMI. Available at: *www.theheart.org/article/821109.do.* Last accessed January 2008.

16.   Rajagopal V, Bhatt DL. Factor Xa inhibitors in acute coronary syndromes: moving from mythology to reality. *J Thromb Haemost* 2005; **3**:426–438.

17.   Cohen M, Bhatt DL, Alexander JH, *et al.* Randomized, double-blind, dose-ranging study of otamixaban, a novel, parenteral, short-acting direct factor Xa inhibitor in percutaneous coronary intervention: the SEPIA-PCI trial. *Circulation* 2007; **115**:2642–2651.

18.   Fifth Organization to Assess Strategies in Acute Ischemic Syndromes Investigators. Comparison of fondaparinux and enoxaparin in acute coronary syndromes. *N Engl J Med* 2006; **354**:1464–1476.

19.   Yusuf S, Mehta SR, Chrolavicius S, *et al.*; OASIS-6 Trial Group. Effects of fondaparinux on mortality and reinfarction in patients with acute ST-segment elevation myocardial infarction. *JAMA* 2006; **295**:1519–1530.

Chapter 7

Miscellaneous therapies

The prior two chapters discussed anti-platelet and anti-thrombin therapies for the treatment of ACS. Together they form the foundation for ACS management, especially during reperfusion therapy. However, other therapies, such as statins, beta-blockers and ACE inhibitors are also important. These therapies not only help to limit infarct size and reduce recurrent myocardial infarction, but also improve survival.

Statins

Statins (HMG-Co-A reductase inhibitors) safely and effectively reduce total cholesterol levels primarily through lowering low-density lipoprotein cholesterol, although they have only recently been thoroughly evaluated in the setting of ACS. The MIRACL (Myocardial Ischemia Reduction with Aggressive Cholesterol Lowering) trial studied the effect of 80 mg of atorvastatin compared with placebo in patients with non-ST-elevation ACS [1]. The investigators concluded that potent lipid-lowering therapy reduced recurrent angina; however, there was no reduction in death or myocardial infarction at 4 months of follow-up. A meta-analysis of similarly designed trials with short-term follow-up in a total of 13,024 patients confirmed that this therapy did not reduce death, myocardial infarction or stroke at 4 months of follow-up [2]. In contrast, an analysis of trials with long-term follow-up in nearly 10,000 patients was able to show that statin therapy initiated during an ACS reduced death, unstable angina and need for revascularization at a mean follow-up of 23 months (*see* Figure 7.1) [3]. Low-density lipoprotein cholesterol was reduced from 132 mg/dL to 86 mg/dL, and only 84 patients needed to be treated with this therapy to prevent one death.

The PROVE-IT (Pravastatin and Atorvastatin Evaluation and Infection Therapy) trial deserves special mention [4]. This trial documented the superiority of atorvastatin 80 mg when compared with pravastatin 40 mg in reducing low-density lipoprotein cholesterol (62 mg/dL versus 95 mg/dL, respectively; $p<0.001$), and adverse cardiovascular events. Accordingly, ACS patients should be started on a statin medication (preferably high-dose atorvastatin) by the time of hospital discharge and use the medication long-term to improve survival. There is some evidence from registry data and small randomized clinical trials that statins initiated early and especially prior to percutaneous

A.A. Bavry, D.L. Bhatt (eds.), *Acute Coronary Syndromes in Clinical Practice*   61
DOI 10.1007/978-1-84800-358-3_7, © Springer-Verlag London Limited 2009

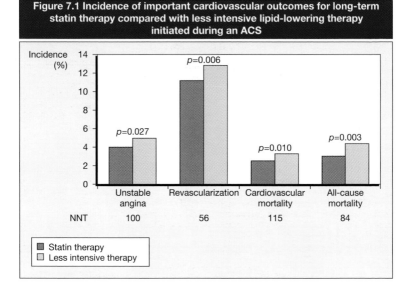

Figure 7.1 Incidence of important cardiovascular outcomes for long-term statin therapy compared with less intensive lipid-lowering therapy initiated during an ACS

NNT, number needed to treat. Reproduced with permission from Bavry *et al.* [3].

coronary intervention reduce ischemic events [5–7]. Potentially, these very early benefits are due to anti-inflammatory effects (*see* Figure 7.2) [8,9].

Angiotensin-converting enzyme inhibitors

ACE inhibitors have been shown to be beneficial to patients with left ventricular dysfunction. They have also been extensively studied during ACS. A meta-analysis of nearly 100,000 patients with acute myocardial infarction documented that ACE inhibitors (mainly captopril) produce an early survival advantage [10]. The absolute benefit derived from ACE inhibitors was greater among high-risk patients. It is recommended that all patients with an ACS receive an oral ACE inhibitor when they are deemed to be hemodynamically stable. The long-term use of these agents will be determined by the presence of high-risk features such as left ventricular dysfunction, diabetes, or renal insufficiency. Angiotensin receptor blockers are a reasonable alternative to patients who are intolerant to ACE inhibitors; however, there is concern of increased adverse events when the two agents are combined [11].

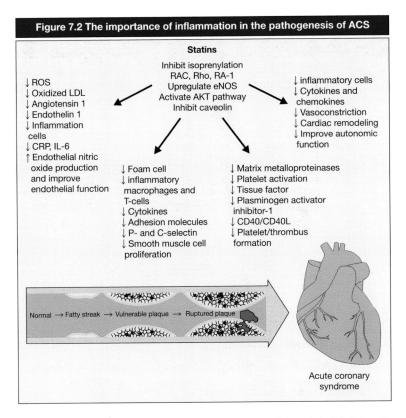

Figure 7.2 The importance of inflammation in the pathogenesis of ACS

AKT, a serine/threonine kinase; CRP, C-reactive protein; eNOS, endothelial nitric oxide synthase; IL-6, interleukin 6; LDL, low-density lipoprotein; RA-1, Rap-activated 1; RAC and Rho, G-protein subunits; ROS, reactive oxygen species. Reproduced with permission from Patel *et al*. [8].

Beta-blockers

Beta-blockers reduce myocardial oxygen demand and contractility. They have been extensively studied in acute myocardial infarction; however, until recently most of the available data pre-dated the reperfusion era. Before mechanical and chemical reperfusion became widespread, the use of intravenous beta-blockers was shown to significantly reduce mortality compared with placebo [12]. An analysis from the early thrombolytic era documented the beneficial effect of beta-blockers, although it also showed that intravenous use was associated with increased mortality, heart failure, shock, and the need for pacemaker placement, compared with oral use [13]. The largest and most recent study conducted on the topic was the COMMIT (ClOpidogrel and Metoprolol in Myocardial Infarction) trial [14]. This mega-trial randomized 45,852 patients with ST-elevation myocardial infarction to either placebo or intravenous then oral metoprolol. Over 50% of the patients received thrombolytic reperfusion therapy. The use of metoprolol decreased the incidence of reinfarction and ventricular fibrillation; however, this came at a cost of increased cardiogenic shock early during admission. This illustrates that beta-blockers are best reserved for use in low-risk acute myocardial infarction patients (*see* Figure 7.3) [14]. Similarly, in ACS patients undergoing percutaneous coronary intervention, the use of beta-blockers has been associated with improved survival [15,16]. In summary, for appropriately selected ACS patients, beta-blockers are beneficial in reducing adverse outcomes. Beta-blockers should not be given until mechanical complications of acute myocardial infarction are ruled out and patients are hemodynamically stable.

Calcium-channel blockers

Short-acting nifedipine has been associated with increased mortality, presumably due to hypotension and reflex tachycardia, and therefore should not be used. Diltiazem or verapamil can be used in special circumstances; however, they have not been shown to improve survival [17]. These agents may be used in patients with ongoing ischemia due to tachyarrhythmia if there is a significant allergy to beta-blockers such as bronchospasm. They may also be useful for coronary spasm.

Nitrates/novel anti-anginal agents

Nitrates have long been used in the care of ACS patients. Despite this, they have not been shown to prevent adverse cardiovascular events [18]. However, in the absence of contraindications, they should be used with the goal of eliminating or reducing symptomatic ischemia, especially during

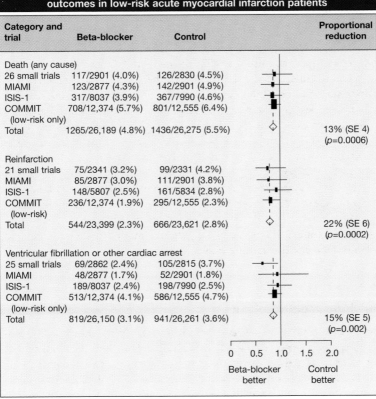

Figure 7.3 Beneficial effect of beta-blockers on important outcomes in low-risk acute myocardial infarction patients

Category and trial	Beta-blocker	Control		Proportional reduction
Death (any cause)				
26 small trials	117/2901 (4.0%)	126/2830 (4.5%)		
MIAMI	123/2877 (4.3%)	142/2901 (4.9%)		
ISIS-1	317/8037 (3.9%)	367/7990 (4.6%)		
COMMIT (low-risk only)	708/12,374 (5.7%)	801/12,555 (6.4%)		
Total	1265/26,189 (4.8%)	1436/26,275 (5.5%)		13% (SE 4) (p=0.0006)
Reinfarction				
21 small trials	75/2341 (3.2%)	99/2331 (4.2%)		
MIAMI	85/2877 (3.0%)	111/2901 (3.8%)		
ISIS-1	148/5807 (2.5%)	161/5834 (2.8%)		
COMMIT (low-risk)	236/12,374 (1.9%)	295/12,555 (2.3%)		
Total	544/23,399 (2.3%)	666/23,621 (2.8%)		22% (SE 6) (p=0.0002)
Ventricular fibrillation or other cardiac arrest				
25 small trials	69/2862 (2.4%)	105/2815 (3.7%)		
MIAMI	48/2877 (1.7%)	52/2901 (1.8%)		
ISIS-1	189/8037 (2.4%)	198/7990 (2.5%)		
COMMIT (low-risk only)	513/12,374 (4.1%)	586/12,555 (4.7%)		
Total	819/26,150 (3.1%)	941/26,261 (3.6%)		15% (SE 5) (p=0.002)

0   0.5   1.0   1.5   2.0

Beta-blocker better   Control better

COMMIT, ClOpidogrel and Metoprolol in Myocardial Infarction Trial; ISIS-1, First International Study of Infarct Survival; MIAMI, metoprolol in acute myocardial infarction. Reproduced with permission from Chen *et al.* [14].

medical stabilization prior to coronary revascularization. Ranolazine is a novel anti-anginal agent (piperazine derivative) that does not cause significant hemodynamic effects. The use of this agent in non-ST-elevation ACS has been shown to safely reduce recurrent ischemia [19]. This agent may serve an important role in optimized acute ACS patients who have persistent ischemic symptoms and marginal hemodynamics.

Summary

In summary, important adjuvant therapy in the care of ACS patients includes statins, ACE inhibitors, and beta-blockers. All of these agents are given with the expectation of improving survival. For ACE inhibitors and beta-blockers, appropriate patient selection is paramount and they should only be administered when hemodynamic stability is assured. ACE inhibitors should be administered orally, as should beta-blockers. Diltiazem or verapamil can be administered selectively, when there is a contraindication to beta-blockers. Nitrates should be used during the medical stabilization of patients with ACS; however, the aim with their use is minimization of ischemia and not a reduction in mortality.

References

1.   Schwartz GG, Olsson AG, Ezekowitz MD, *et al*. Effects of atorvastatin on early recurrent ischemic events in acute coronary syndromes. The MIRACL study: a randomized controlled trial. *JAMA* 2001; **285**:1711–1718.

2.   Briel M, Schwartz GG, Thompson PL, *et al*. Effects of early treatment with statins on short-term clinical outcomes in acute coronary syndromes: a meta-analysis of randomized controlled trials. *JAMA* 2006; **295**:2046–2056.

3.   Bavry AA, Mood GR, Kumbhani DJ, *et al*. Long-term benefit of statin therapy initiated during the hospitalization for an acute coronary syndrome: a systematic review of randomized trials. *Am J Cardiovasc Drugs* 2007; **7**:135–141.

4.   Cannon CP, Braunwald E, McCabe CH, *et al*. Intensive versus moderate lipid lowering with statins after acute coronary syndromes. *NEJM* 2004; **350**:1495–1504.

5.   Chan AW, Bhatt DL, Chew DP, *et al*. Early and sustained survival benefit associated with statin therapy at the time of percutaneous coronary intervention. *Circulation* 2002; **105**:691–696.

6.   Chan AW, Bhatt DL, Chew DP, et al. Relation of inflammation and benefit of statins after percutaneous coronary interventions. *Circulation* 2003; **107**:1750–1756.

7.   Patti G, Pasceri V, Colonna G, *et al*. Atorvastatin pretreatment improves outcomes in patients with acute coronary syndromes undergoing early percutaneous coronary intervention: results of the ARMYDA-ACS randomized trial. *J Am Coll Cardiol* 2007; **49**:1272–1278.

8.   Patel TN, Shishehbor MH, Bhatt DL. A review of high-dose statin therapy: targeting cholesterol and inflammation in atherosclerosis. *Eur Heart J* 2007; **28**:664–672.

9.   Shishehbor MH, Patel TN, Bhatt DL. Using statins to treat inflammation in acute coronary syndromes: are we there yet? *Cleve Clin J Med* 2006; **73**:760–766.

10.   Indications for ACE inhibitors in the early treatment of acute myocardial infarction: systematic overview of individual data from 100,000 patients in randomized trials. ACE Inhibitor Myocardial Infarction Collaborative Group. *Circulation* 1998; **97**:2202–2212.

11. Pfeffer MA, McMurray JJ, Velazquez EJ, *et al*. Valsartan, captopril, or both in myocardial infarction complicated by heart failure, left ventricular dysfunction, or both. *N Engl J Med* 2003; **349**:1893–1906.

12. Freemantle N, Cleland J, Young P, *et al*. Beta blockade after myocardial infarction: systematic review and meta regression analysis. *BMJ* 1999; **318**:1730–1737.

13. Pfisterer M, Cox JL, Granger CB, *et al*. Atenolol use and clinical outcomes after thrombolysis for acute myocardial infarction: the GUSTO-I experience. Global Utilization of Streptokinase and TPA (alteplase) for Occluded Coronary Arteries. *J Am Coll Cardiol* 1998; **32**:634–640.

14. Chen ZM, Pan HC, Chen YP, *et al*.; COMMIT (ClOpidogrel and Metoprolol in Myocardial Infarction Trial) collaborative group. Early intravenous then oral metoprolol in 45,852 patients with acute myocardial infarction: randomised placebo-controlled trial. *Lancet* 2005; **366**:1622–1632.

15. Ellis K, Tcheng JE, Sapp S, *et al*. Mortality benefit of beta blockade in patients with acute coronary syndromes undergoing coronary intervention: pooled results from the Epic, Epilog, Epistent, Capture and Rapport Trials. *J Interv Cardiol* 2003; **16**:299–305.

16. Chan AW, Quinn MJ, Bhatt DL, *et al*. Mortality benefit of beta-blockade after successful elective percutaneous coronary intervention. *J Am Coll Cardiol* 2002; **40**:669–675.

17. The effect of diltiazem on mortality and reinfarction after myocardial infarction. The Multicenter Diltiazem Postinfarction Trial Research Group. *N Engl J Med* 1988; **319**:385–392.

18. ISIS-4: a randomised factorial trial assessing early oral captopril, oral mononitrate, and intravenous magnesium sulphate in 58,050 patients with suspected acute myocardial infarction. ISIS-4 (Fourth International Study of Infarct Survival) Collaborative Group. *Lancet* 1995; **345**:669–685.

19. Morrow DA, Scirica BM, Karwatowska-Prokopczuk E, *et al*. Effects of ranolazine on recurrent cardiovascular events in patients with non-ST-elevation acute coronary syndromes. The MERLIN-TIMI 36 randomized trial. *JAMA* 2007; **297**:1775–1783.

Chapter 8

Revascularization and reperfusion therapy

This chapter focuses on revascularization and reperfusion therapy in the setting of ACS. Revascularization therapy is distinct from reperfusion therapy. The former takes place in non-ST-elevation or ST-elevation ACS, while reperfusion is employed only for ST-elevation myocardial infarction. Revascularization therapy for non-ST-elevation ACS is usually considered an urgent condition unless there are signs of hemodynamic or electrical instability, in which case it is performed immediately. Instability in these patients may indicate a large burden of jeopardized myocardium or rather a disguised ST-elevation myocardial infarction, which, for example, can be seen with a circumflex artery occlusion. In contrast, reperfusion therapy is an emergent condition since it characterizes a state of coronary occlusion. A small subset of non-ST-elevation myocardial infarction patients will only receive medical therapy, even after coronary angiography. Revascularization is usually accomplished percutaneously, although some of these patients will be referred for surgical revascularization. While thrombolytic therapy is contraindicated for non-ST-elevation myocardial infarction, it has an important role in ST-elevation myocardial infarction when primary angioplasty is not readily available. Our discussion will begin with revascularization therapy and then move into reperfusion therapy.

Revascularization therapy

The role of revascularization therapy versus initial medical management for non-ST-elevation ACS has been somewhat controversial. One of the largest and earliest trials on the topic was the VANQWISH (Veterans Affairs Non-Q-Wave Infarction Strategies in Hospital) trial published in 1998 [1]. This trial randomized 920 patients within 72 hours of the onset of chest pain to a strategy of invasive therapy and appropriate revascularization versus initial medical management. Patients in the medical arm could cross-over to an invasive strategy if a large burden of ischemia was demonstrated on stress testing, or they demonstrated hemodynamic or electrical instability during their hospital course. From hospital discharge until 1 year of follow-up there were significantly more deaths with the invasive strategy; however,

A.A. Bavry, D.L. Bhatt (eds.), Acute Coronary Syndromes in Clinical Practice   69
DOI 10.1007/978-1-84800-358-3_8, © Springer-Verlag London Limited 2009

there were similar deaths at the extent of follow-up (44 months) (*see* Figure 8.1) [1]. Unfortunately, this trial was conducted prior to the availability of glycoprotein IIb/IIIa inhibitors and intra-coronary stents, which could have unfavorably biased the invasive group.

A more contemporary trial was the TACTICS-TIMI 18 (Treat Angina with Aggrastat and Determine Cost of Therapy with an Invasive or Conservative Strategy-Thrombolysis in Myocardial Infarction) trial [2]. This trial randomized 2220 patients with non-ST-elevation ACS to a similar invasive versus conservative strategy. This trial is notable in that, by design, all participants received tirofiban for 48 hours or until revascularization, and stents were used in more than 80% of percutaneous coronary interventions. Patients in the invasive arm underwent coronary angiography a median of 22 hours after randomization. Unlike VANQWISH, this trial documented a significant reduction in the composite outcome of death, nonfatal myocardial

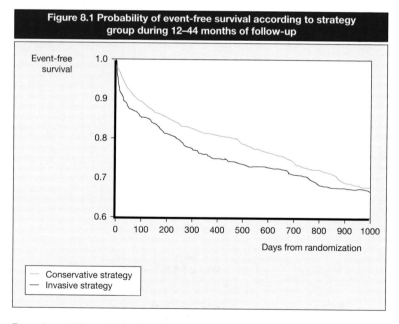

Figure 8.1 Probability of event-free survival according to strategy group during 12–44 months of follow-up

Reproduced with permission from Boden *et al.* [1].

infarction and rehospitalization for unstable angina at 6 months of follow-up. The benefit of invasive therapy appeared to be most pronounced for patients with an intermediate or higher TIMI risk score (*see* Figure 8.2) [2]. Invasive therapy did not reduce ischemic events in low-risk patients, although it was still a cost-effective approach.

Figure 8.2 Benefit of invasive therapy is more pronounced for patients with an intermediate or higher TIMI risk score

Baseline variable	Number (%)	Odds ratio	Primary end point	
			Invasive strategy	Conservative strategy
Age <65 years	1258 (57)		14.9	17.8
Age ≥65 years	962 (43)		17.1	21.7
Men	1463 (66)		15.3	19.4
Women	757 (34)		17.0	19.6
Prior MI	866 (39)		18.8	24.2
No prior MI	1354 (61)		14.0	16.4
Prior aspirin use	1477 (66)		17.7	18.6
No prior aspirin use	743 (34)		12.2	21.0
Diabetes	613 (28)		20.1	27.7
No diabetes	1607 (72)		14.2	16.4
ST-segment changes	852 (38)		16.4	26.3
No ST-segment changes	1368 (62)		15.6	15.3
CK-MB >5 ng/mL	833 (39)		17.3	23.9
CK-MB ≤5 ng/mL	1297 (61)		15.4	16.8
Troponin T >0.1 ng/mL	748 (43)		16.4	24.5
Troponin T ≤0.1 ng/mL	1078 (59)		15.1	16.6
TIMI risk score				
0–2 (low)	555 (25)		12.8	11.8
3–4 (intermediate)	1328 (60)		16.1	20.3
5–7 (high)	337 (15)		19.5	30.6

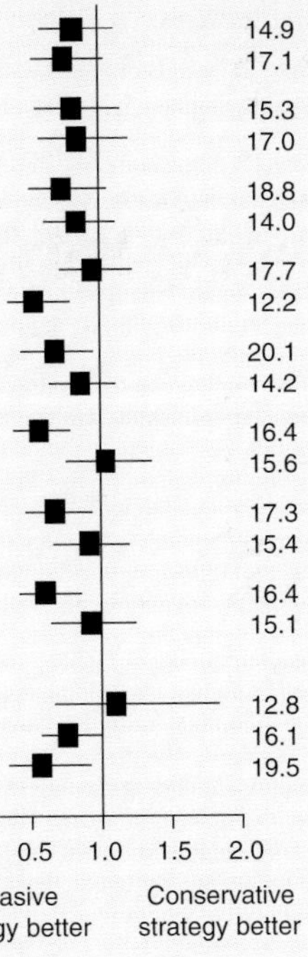

0   0.5   1.0   1.5   2.0

Invasive strategy better   Conservative strategy better

CK-MB, creatine kinase myocardial band isoenzyme; MI, myocardial infarction; TIMI, Thrombolysis in Myocardial Infarction. Reproduced with permission from Cannon *et al.* [2].

The most recent trial on the topic is the ICTUS (Invasive Versus Conservative Treatment in Unstable Coronary Syndromes Investigators) trial, which studied 1200 troponin-positive patients [3]. Although the TACTICS-TIMI 18 trial was contemporary, an aim of the ICTUS trial was to provide optimal medical therapy (e.g., enoxaparin, statins, and clopidogrel) to all conservatively managed patients. There was no demonstrable benefit to routine invasive therapy at 1–3 years of follow-up. Moreover, there was significantly more myocardial infarction among recipients of early invasive therapy, although the excess was due to higher rates of peri-procedural myocardial infarction, the prognostic significance of which is less than *de novo* myocardial infarction. Part of the explanation for these findings may be due to the fact that more than 50% of conservative patients eventually underwent revascularization during the extent of follow-up, compared to nearly 80% of invasive patients. Another explanation is the significant degree of benefit provided by optimal medical therapy. This trial illustrates that troponin status alone may not be a sufficient mechanism to risk stratify patients, and more sophisticated risk scores are needed to determine the highest risk patients. Another point is that low-risk patients are expected to do well with optimal conservative therapy. This is consistent with an earlier meta-analysis that documented a significant benefit among men who received invasive therapy [4]. Unfortunately, the same was not true for women as there was no obvious benefit in this group (*see* Figure 8.3). Women often have less severe coronary disease than men and more potential for procedural complications. Therefore, appropriate risk stratification, including the use of troponins, is particularly important to select women who may benefit from an invasive strategy [5,6].

A meta-analysis of contemporary trials containing a total of 8375 patients, and including the TACTICS-TIMI 18 and ICTUS trials, documented that invasive therapy results in a 25% reduction in mortality and a 17% reduction in myocardial infarction during a mean follow-up of 2 years [7]. Invasive therapy also results in fewer rehospitalizations for unstable angina. A concern among the individual trials is that a large proportion of conservatively managed patients crossed over to invasive therapy, such as the ICTUS trial, thus attenuating any potential benefit from invasive therapy. This meta-analysis attempted to adjust for this limitation. Trials were grouped together that most retained their original study design (i.e., few conservative patients crossed over to invasive therapy), and compared

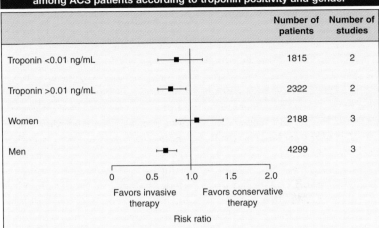

Figure 8.3 Effect of invasive therapy versus conservative therapy among ACS patients according to troponin positivity and gender

		Number of patients	Number of studies
Troponin <0.01 ng/mL		1815	2
Troponin >0.01 ng/mL		2322	2
Women		2188	3
Men		4299	3

Reproduced with permission from Bavry *et al.* [4].

them to studies where a large proportion of conservative patients crossed over to invasive therapy. This revealed that a large difference in the use of revascularization between treatment arms and not the time to angiography was a significant factor in determining the beneficial effect of early invasive therapy (*see* Figure 8.4) [7].

In summary, invasive therapy with appropriate revascularization remains beneficial in the treatment of non-ST-elevation ACS as illustrated by registry data and meta-analyses (*see* Figure 4.6) [4,7–10]. Current guidelines place emphasis on risk stratification for patients with ACS [11,12]. Risk assessment should be comprehensive, rather than just a determination of troponin positivity or dynamic electrocardiographic changes. The goal in the management of ACS is to direct the highest risk patients to invasive therapy with the expectation to improve survival and reduce myocardial infarction. Conservative and optimal medical therapy should be preferential for the lowest risk patients.

Approximately 10% of non-ST-elevation ACS patients will be referred for coronary artery bypass grafting due to severe left main artery disease,

Figure 8.4 Role of time to angiography and extent of revascularization in determining the benefit of early invasive therapy

Characteristic		Relative risk reduction (%)	p-value	Number of patients
Angiography <24 hours		18	0.26	3961
Angiography ≥24 hours		27	0.002	4414
Small difference in revascularization betwen treatment arms		12	0.55	2630
Intermediate difference in revascularization between treatment arms		22	0.03	3158
Large difference in revascularization between treatment arms		37	0.01	2587

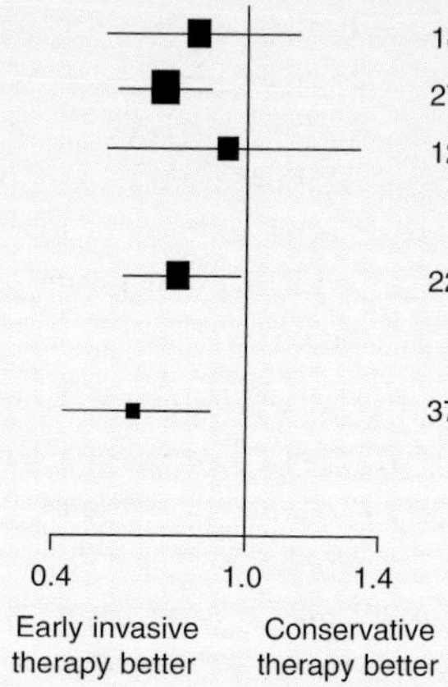

0.4   1.0   1.4

Early invasive   Conservative
therapy better   therapy better

Results show that the rate of revascularization among patients with ACS and not time to angiography is a significant determinant of the benefit of invasive therapy. Reproduced with permission from Bavry et al. [7].

severe diffuse multi-vessel coronary disease, or other causes, while 20% of patients will undergo medical management without revascularization for a variety of reasons [13]. Therefore, approximately two-thirds of patients with ACS will undergo percutaneous coronary intervention.

Drug-eluting stents were initially studied in stable patients. As the penetration of these devices increased, their use in relatively nontested populations such as ACS also increased [14]. Several trials have now reported the use of drug-eluting stents in ACS [15]. While this analysis documented the benefit of drug-eluting stents in this population, important safety questions remain [16]. A high proportion of ACS patients have been documented to self-terminate their clopidogrel, which is associated with increased mortality [17]. Until further safety data are accumulated, the use of a bare-metal stent in an ACS should be preferential [18].

Reperfusion therapy

Although thrombolytic therapy is contraindicated in non-ST-elevation ACS, this constitutes the majority of reperfusion therapy for ST-elevation myocardial infarction worldwide. Thrombolysis saves 30 lives for every 1000 patients treated within 6 hours of chest pain onset and 20 lives for every 1000 patients treated 7–12 hours after chest pain [19]. This forms the basis of the recommendation that thrombolytic therapy should be given to individuals without a contraindication to its use within 12 hours, although preferably within 6 hours. Although thrombolysis is unequivocally life saving, coronary flow is not restored in 15% of patients and at least 1% may experience intracranial hemorrhage [20,21].

Primary angioplasty is superior to thrombolysis in reducing mortality, myocardial infarction, and stoke [22]. In fact, primary angioplasty results in a 2% absolute reduction in mortality compared with thrombolysis, irrespective of the type of lytic agent used. Unfortunately, the worldwide availability of primary angioplasty is limited. This led to attempts to combine the ease and availability of thrombolysis with angioplasty through so called 'facilitated percutaneous coronary intervention'. The result of this strategy has been universally disappointing as it results in excess mortality, myocardial infarction, stroke, and major bleeding when compared with primary angioplasty [23]. Therefore, a patient who has received thrombolytic therapy should not undergo angioplasty unless there is evidence of failure of lysis, which is termed 'rescue percutaneous coronary intervention' [24,25]. This strategy improves survival compared with conservative therapy.

Summary

In summary, revascularization for non-ST-elevation ACS and reperfusion for ST-elevation myocardial infarction saves lives. Revascularization is preferred to conservative therapy among moderate- and high-risk individuals, although low-risk patients can be initially managed with optimal medical therapy. Thrombolysis forms the foundation of reperfusion therapy, although primary angioplasty is preferable when it is readily available. Patients who successfully receive thrombolysis should undergo further risk-stratification through stress testing and assessment of left ventricular function to determine the need for additional revascularization, although patients who fail thrombolysis should be promptly referred for angioplasty.

References

1.   Boden WE, O'Rourke RA, Crawford MH, *et al*. Outcomes in patients with acute non-Q-wave myocardial infarction randomly assigned to an invasive as compared with a conservative management strategy. Veterans Affairs Non-Q-Wave Infarction Strategies in Hospital (VANQWISH) Trial Investigators. *N Engl J Med* 1998; **338**:1785–1792.

2.   Cannon CP, Weintraub WS, Demopoulos LA, *et al*.; TACTICS (Treat Angina with Aggrastat and Determine Cost of Therapy with an Invasive or Conservative Strategy) – Thrombolysis in Myocardial Infarction 18 Investigators. Comparison of early invasive and conservative strategies in patients with unstable coronary syndromes treated with glycoprotein IIb/IIIa inhibitor tirofiban. *N Engl J Med* 2001; **344**:1879–1887.

3.   de Winter RJ, Windhausen F, Cornel JH, *et al*. Early invasive versus selectively invasive management for acute coronary syndromes. *N Engl J Med* 2005; **353**:1095–1104.

4.   Bavry AA, Kumbhani DJ, Quiroz R, *et al*. Invasive therapy along with glycoprotein IIb/IIIa inhibitors and intracoronary stents improves survival in non-ST segment elevation acute coronary syndromes: a meta-analysis and review of the literature. *Am J Cardiol* 2004; **93**:830–835.

5.   Hochman JS, McCabe CH, Stone PH, *et al*. Outcome and profile of women and men presenting with acute coronary syndromes: a report from TIMI IIIB. TIMI Investigators. Thrombolysis in Myocardial Infarction. *J Am Coll Cardiol* 1997; **30**:141–148.

6.   Clayton TC, Pocock SJ, Henderson RA, *et al*. Do men benefit more than women from an interventional strategy in patients with unstable angina or non-ST-elevation myocardial infarction? The impact of gender in the RITA 3 trial. *Eur Heart J* 2004; **25**:1641–1650.

7.   Bavry AA, Kumbhani DJ, Rassi AN, *et al*. Benefit of early invasive therapy in acute coronary syndromes a meta-analysis of contemporary randomized clinical trials. *J Am Coll Cardiol* 2006; **48**:1319–1325.

8.   Mehta SR, Cannon CP, Fox KA, *et al*. Routine vs selective invasive strategies in patients with acute coronary syndromes: a collaborative meta-analysis of randomized trials. *JAMA* 2005; **293**:2908–2917.

9.   Bhatt DL. To cath or not to cath: that is no longer the question. *JAMA* 2005; **293**:2935–2937.

10.   Bhatt DL, Roe MT, Peterson ED, *et al*. Utilization of early invasive management strategies for high-risk patients with non-ST-segment elevation acute coronary syndromes. Results from the CRUSADE quality improvement initiative. *JAMA* 2004; **292**:2096–2104.

11.   Anderson JL, Adams CD, Antman EM, *et al*. ACC/AHA 2007 Guidelines for the Management of Patients With Unstable Angina/Non–ST-Elevation Myocardial Infarction—Executive Summary. *J Am Coll Cardiol* 2007; **50**:652–726.

12.   Bassand JP, Hamm CW, Ardissino D, *et al*. Guidelines for the diagnosis and treatment of non-ST-segment elevation acute coronary syndromes. The task force for the diagnosis and treatment of non-ST-segment elevation acute coronary syndromes of the European Society of Cardiology. *Eur Heart J* 2007; **28**:1598–1660.

13. Ferguson JJ, Califf RM, Antman EM, *et al*. Enoxaparin vs unfractionated heparin in high-risk patients with non-ST-segment elevation acute coronary syndromes managed with an intended early invasive strategy: primary results of the SYNERGY randomized trial. *JAMA* 2004; **292**:45–54.

14. Kandzari DE, Roe MT, Ohman EM, *et al*. Frequency, predictors, and outcomes of drug-eluting stent utilization in patients with high-risk non-ST-segment elevation acute coronary syndromes. *Am J Cardiol* 2005; **96**:750–755.

15. Pasceri V, Patti G, Speciale G, *et al*. Meta-analysis of clinical trials on use of drug eluting stents for treatment of acute myocardial infarction. *Am Heart J* 2007; **153**:749–754.

16. Bavry AA, Bhatt DL. Acute myocardial infarction and drug-eluting stents: a green light for their use or time for measured restraint? *Am Heart J* 2007; **153**:719–721.

17. Spertus JA, Kettelkamp R, Vance C, *et al*. Prevalence, predictors, and outcomes of premature discontinuation of thienopyridine therapy after drug-eluting stent placement: results from the PREMIER registry. *Circulation* 2006; **113**:2803–2809.

18. Bavry AA, Bhatt DL. Drug-eluting stents: dual antiplatelet therapy for every survivor? *Circulation* 2007; **116**:696–699.

19. Fibrinolytic Therapy Trialists' Collaborative Group. Indications for fibrinolytic therapy in suspected acute myocardial infarction: collaborative overview of early mortality and major morbidity results from all randomized trials of more than 1,000 patients. *Lancet* 1994; **343**:311–322.

20. The GUSTO Angiographic Investigators. The effect of tissue plasminogen activator, streptokinase, or both on coronary-artery patency, ventricular function, and survival after acute myocardial infarction. *N Engl J Med* 1993; **329**:1615–1622.

21. Keeley EC, Grines CL. Primary coronary intervention for acute myocardial infarction. *JAMA* 2004; **291**:736–739.

22. Keeley EC, Grines CL. Primary angioplasty versus intravenous thrombolytic therapy for acute myocardial infarction: a quantitative review of 23 randomised trials. *Lancet* 2003; **361**:13–20.

23. Keeley EC, Boura JA, Grines CL. Comparison of primary and facilitated percutaneous coronary interventions for ST-elevation myocardial infarction: quantitative review of randomized trials. *Lancet* 2006; **367**:579–588.

24. Patel TN, Bavry AA, Kumbhani DJ, *et al*. A meta-analysis of randomized trials of rescue percutaneous coronary intervention after failed fibrinolysis. *Am J Cardiol* 2006; **97**:1685–1690.

25. Gershlick AH, Stephens-Lloyd A, Hughes S, *et al*. Rescue angioplasty after failed thrombolytic therapy for acute myocardial infarction. *N Engl J Med* 2005; **353**:2758–2768.

Chapter 9

Controversies and future approaches

Cardiology is a rapidly moving field that has recently seen significant medical and invasive advances. This has resulted in improved patient outcomes. While this is good, we are reminded that there are numerous areas in the management of ACS that remain somewhat controversial or unsettled. This uncertainty in the optimal management of unstable coronary patients is a fertile area for continued debate and future research. In this chapter, the first area of discussion is optimal reperfusion therapy for ST-elevation myocardial infarction, followed by optimal revascularization for non-ST-elevation myocardial infarction. The last section touches upon future approaches to the management of cardiovascular disease.

Facilitated percutaneous coronary intervention

One area that has been reasonably well resolved is the issue of facilitated percutaneous coronary intervention (*see* Chapter 8). This approach seemed promising given the ease of administering thrombolytic therapy coupled to the superiority of angioplasty. However, a large meta-analysis documented that percutaneous coronary intervention facilitated by full-dose thrombolytic agents is deleterious [1]. Although this approach increased initial TIMI 3 flow, there was also increased mortality, myocardial infarction, stroke, subsequent revascularization, and major bleeding.

There were relatively few studies in the meta-analysis that addressed percutaneous coronary intervention facilitated by half-dose thrombolytics and a glycoprotein IIb/IIIa inhibitor. The FINESSE (Facilitated Intervention with Enhanced Reperfusion Speed to Stop Events) trial was recently reported at the European Society for Cardiology meeting and helped to fill this gap in knowledge [2]. The trial randomized 2452 patients to one of the following arms:

- primary angioplasty;
- abciximab-facilitated intervention;
- half-dose reteplase and abciximab-facilitated intervention.

A.A. Bavry, D.L. Bhatt (eds.), Acute Coronary Syndromes in Clinical Practice
DOI 10.1007/978-1-84800-358-3_9, © Springer-Verlag London Limited 2009

The facilitated arms had no reduction in the composite end point, although major bleeding was increased with a trend toward increased intra-cranial hemorrhage.

In summary, while thrombolytic therapy is beneficial and should continue to be used globally where there is a lack of primary angioplasty centers, a large body of evidence strongly cautions against performing coronary intervention facilitated with either full- or half-dose thrombolytics. Patients who receive thrombolytics should be conservatively treated and undergo risk stratification unless there is evidence of failure of lysis [3].

The optimal time to wait before performing coronary intervention if high-risk features are identified (such as documentation of left ventricular dysfunction or a significant burden of ischemia by stress testing) is controversial. A minimum delay between lysis and angioplasty of 48–72 hours would seem reasonable. If there is ongoing chest discomfort after thrombolysis, rescue percutaneous coronary intervention is strongly indicated [4].

Early invasive versus conservative management

In non-ST-elevation myocardial infarction, the issue of early invasive therapy versus conservative management seems to be a moving target. Older trials documented harm from early invasive therapy [5], whereas more contemporary trials documented benefit from this approach [6], and the most recent trial seemed to be neutral [7]. Unfortunately, in the recent ICTUS (Invasive Versus Conservative Treatment in Unstable Coronary Syndromes Investigators) trial, a large number of patients crossed over from conservative to invasive therapy. This diluted the ability to test the trial's hypothesis, since a large proportion of both patients received invasive therapy during the extent of follow-up (*see* Figure 8.4) [8]. In contrast, trials that retain more of the original randomization scheme display significant benefit from early invasive therapy. Another point is that invasive therapy has become much safer since the earliest trials, due to the introduction of advanced anti-thrombotics and stents. Similarly, medical therapy has markedly improved with the use of thienopyridines and statins, which were widely used in conservatively treated patients in the ICTUS trial.

The most recent cardiology guidelines highlight that risk stratification should be emphasized for patients with non-ST-elevation ACS [9]. For example, low-risk non-ST-elevation myocardial infarction patients may be preferentially treated conservatively, while high-risk patients should continue to receive invasive therapy. The other point is that troponin status alone may not be sufficient to identify high-risk patients, and that the degree of troponin elevation and the use of risk models may be more sensitive.

Culprit-vessel versus multi-vessel intervention

Currently, multi-vessel coronary intervention is not indicated at the time of an ACS unless there is evidence of cardiogenic shock. Arguments in favor of culprit-vessel-only intervention include the minimization of radiation and contrast, and avoidance of stenting in a thrombotic milieu that could increase the risk for stent thrombosis [10]. In contrast, multi-vessel intervention could reduce exposure to the small but inherent risk of repeat coronary intervention and might also reduce future myocardial infarction by treating additional vulnerable plaques. No randomized trial has addressed this issue, although several registries have [11,12]. The largest study to date reported that this approach significantly reduced the need for subsequent revascularization, although there was a neutral effect on death and myocardial infarction (*see* Figure 9.1) [11]. Until there are randomized trial data, however, this approach should continue to be individualized.

Drug-eluting stents versus bare-metal stents

No recent topic in interventional cardiology has garnered as much attention as drug-eluting stents. The use of drug-eluting stents exploded after their clinical introduction and they quickly represented 80–90% of stent-based procedures [13]. A significant proportion of this use was in untested or 'off-label' indications. While effective in reducing target lesion revascularization [14], drug-eluting stents have been shown to increase the risk for late stent thrombosis [15,16]. This caused the use of drug-eluting stents to decrease in many interventional cardiology laboratories [17].

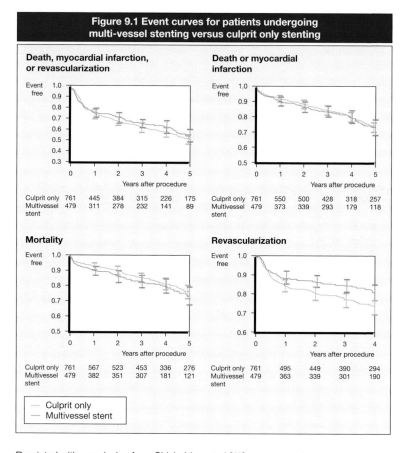

Figure 9.1 Event curves for patients undergoing multi-vessel stenting versus culprit only stenting

Reprinted with permission from Shishehbor *et al.* [11].

Drug-eluting stents have been studied relatively infrequently and with limited follow-up in the setting of acute myocardial infarction. This is a cause of concern since stent implantation during an ACS has been associated with late stent thrombosis [10]. Also, a high proportion of acute myocardial infarction patients have been found to be noncompliant with clopidogrel during follow-up [18]. Therefore, the routine use of drug-eluting stents during emergent ST-elevation ACS should likely be discouraged [19]. Implantation of a drug-eluting stent requires long-term use of dual anti-platelet therapy; therefore, patients should be screened for a high likelihood of compliance to these medications prior to stent implantation. Patients should also be assessed for bleeding risk and the need for future surgical procedures that would require terminating anti-platelet therapy [20]. These issues may be difficult to assess completely if the first meeting with the patient occurs in the catheterization laboratory. In summary, the use of drug-eluting stents in ACS may be problematic due to the limited time to assess a patient's compliance, bleeding risk, and need for future surgical procedures (*see* Figures 9.2 and 9.3) [17,20]. This

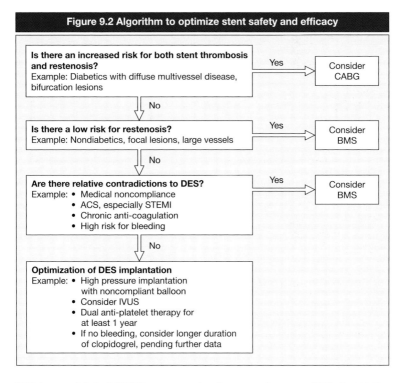

Figure 9.2 Algorithm to optimize stent safety and efficacy

BMS, bare-metal stent; CABG, coronary artery bypass graft surgery; DES, drug-eluting stent; IVUS, intravascular ultrasound; STEMI, ST-elevation myocardial infarction. Reprinted with permission from Bavry *et al.* [17].

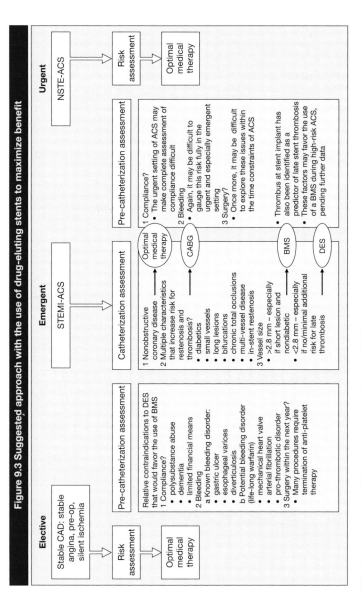

Figure 9.3 Suggested approach with the use of drug-eluting stents to maximize benefit

BMS, bare-metal stent; CAD, coronary artery disease; CABG, coronary artery bypass grafting; DES, drug-eluting stent; NSTEMI, non-ST-elevation myocardial infarction; STEMI, ST-elevation myocardial infarction. Reproduced from Bavry & Bhatt [20].

may favor the use of a bare-metal stent in this population until further data are accumulated.

Unresolved issues include how to manage patients who have a drug-eluting stent and then require surgery, how long clopidogrel should be continued after stent implantation, and what the proper use of drug-eluting stents in 'off-label' patients should be.

Future approaches

The most commonly used, although least studied, anti-thrombin agent in the management of ACS is unfractionated heparin. Despite the efficacy of heparin, it has significant limitations, including life-threatening allergic reactions in a minority of patients. Data on direct thrombin inhibitors are accumulating, as well as Factor Xa inhibitors. Factor Xa is the point at which the extrinsic and intrinsic pathways meet. The goal of these latter two classes of agents is to improve anti-thrombotic efficacy with a more favorable safety profile.

The indirect Factor Xa inhibitor fondaparinux has been studied in the setting of non-ST-elevation and ST-elevation ACS [21,22]. This agent has an improved safety profile compared with low-molecular-weight heparin (i.e., less bleeding), although there are concerns about a lack of efficacy during percutaneous coronary intervention (i.e., catheter-related thrombosis). Direct Factor X inhibitors are also being studied, which will hopefully achieve a more optimal balance of safety and efficacy that may be lacking with the indirect inhibitors [23,24].

The same problems exist with anti-platelet agents of which aspirin is the prototypical agent. Resistance (or relative lack of effect) is commonly discussed and bleeding problems are not infrequent. The imperfections of aspirin lead to the development of the thienopyridines (i.e., ticlopidine and clopidogrel). While these agents appear to be more effective than aspirin, a significant proportion of patients treated with clopidogrel still have low levels of platelet inhibition. Moreover, clopidogrel is irreversible, which makes its use prior to coronary artery bypass grafting potentially problematic. Reversible nonthienopyridines (i.e., the oral agent AZD 6140 or the intravenous cangrelor) are at various stages of development and have the potential to fill this void in currently available anti-platelet agents [25,26].

Numerous technological advances are on the horizon that will allow for more precise and rapid diagnosis of cardiovascular diseases. Chest pain is a heterogeneous diagnosis that is common in the emergency department. Due to the potential for significant downside, emergency room physicians understandably have a low threshold to admit chest pain patients to the hospital. This burdens the healthcare system by resulting in unnecessary hospital stays and costs. The 64-slice multi-detector computed tomography is being investigated as a tool to more rapidly and precisely diagnose chest pain patients. The appeal of this test is that multiple life-threatening diagnoses, such as pulmonary embolus, aortic dissection, and myocardial infarction, can be simultaneously ruled out [27]. As this technology becomes more common, the added harm from the additional radiation and contrast will need to be carefully considered.

With currently available drugs and devices, it is not uncommon that several hundred patients will need to be treated so that one patient will not suffer an adverse outcome such as myocardial infarction or death. This means that an excess of patients take medication or receive a device with potential side-effects (i.e., no benefit) from its use. In the future, pharmacogenomics may play an important role by directing therapy to those most likely to benefit. Angiogenesis and myogenesis may also be important as complementary therapies in the management of ACS. These technologies can also be directed to catheter-based therapies.

Summary

In summary, we have come a long way in a relatively short period of time in managing ACS. Historically, death rates from this disease have declined over the last several decades, although mortality remains high. As treatment questions arise, research has tried to address these important gaps in knowledge. Despite this progress, there are still areas where improvements can be made in the care of cardiovascular patients. The future will likely be characterized by enhanced risk stratification, more effective and safer anti-platelet and anti-thrombin medications, and expanding use of genomic- and pharmacogenomic-based therapy.

References

1.   Keeley EC, Boura JA, Grines CL. Comparison of primary and facilitated percutaneous coronary interventions for ST-elevation myocardial infarction: quantitative review of randomized trials. *Lancet* 2006; **367**:579–588.

2.   FINESSE: Abciximab-only- and lytic/abciximab-facilitated PCI no better than primary PCI. Available at: *www.theheart.org/article/809837.do*. Last accessed December 2007.

3.   Patel TN, Bavry AA, Kumbhani DJ, *et al*. A meta-analysis of randomized trials of rescue percutaneous coronary intervention after failed fibrinolysis. *Am J Cardiol* 2006; **97**:1685–1690.

4.   Gershlick AH, Stephens-Lloyd A, Hughes S, *et al*. Rescue angioplasty after failed thrombolytic therapy for acute myocardial infarction. *N Engl J Med* 2005; **353**:2758–2768.

5.   Boden WE, O'Rourke RA, Crawford MH, *et al*. Outcomes in patients with acute non-Q-wave myocardial infarction randomly assigned to an invasive as compared with a conservative management strategy. Veterans Affairs Non-Q-Wave Infarction Strategies in Hospital (VANQWISH) Trial Investigators. *N Engl J Med* 1998; **338**:1785–1792. Erratum in: *N Engl J Med* 1998; **339**:1091.

6.   Cannon CP, Weintraub WS, Demopoulos LA, *et al*.; TACTICS (Treat Angina with Aggrastat and Determine Cost of Therapy with an Invasive or Conservative Strategy)–Thrombolysis in Myocardial Infarction 18 Investigators. Comparison of early invasive and conservative strategies in patients with unstable coronary syndromes treated with glycoprotein IIb/IIIa inhibitor tirofiban. *N Engl J Med* 2001; **344**:1879–1887.

7.   de Winter RJ, Windhausen F, Cornel JH, *et al*. Early invasive versus selectively invasive management for acute coronary syndromes. *N Engl J Med* 2005; **353**:1095–1104.

8.   Bavry AA, Kumbhani DJ, Rassi AN, *et al*. Benefit of early invasive therapy in acute coronary syndromes a meta-analysis of contemporary randomized clinical trials. *J Am Coll Cardiol* 2006; **48**:1319–1325.

9.   Anderson JL, Adams CD, Antman EM, *et al*. ACC/AHA 2007 guidelines for the management of patients with unstable angina/non ST-elevation myocardial infarction: executive summary. A report of the American College of Cardiology/American Heart Association Task Force on practice guidelines (writing committee to revise the 2002 guidelines for the management of patients with unstable angina/non ST-elevation myocardial infarction. *Circulation* 2007; **116**:803–877.

10.   Daemen J, Wenaweser P, Tsuchida K, *et al*. Early and late coronary stent thrombosis of sirolimus-eluting and paclitaxel-eluting stents in routine clinical practice: data from a large two-institutional cohort study. *Lancet* 2007; **369**:667–678.

11.   Shishehbor MH, Lauer MS, Singh IM, *et al*. In unstable angina or non-ST-segment acute coronary syndrome, should patients with multivessel coronary artery disease undergo multivessel or culprit-only stenting? *J Am Coll Cardiol* 2007; **49**:849–854.

12.   Brener SJ, Murphy SA, Gibson CM, *et al*. Efficacy and safety of multivessel percutaneous revascularization and tirofiban therapy in patients with acute coronary syndromes. *Am J Cardiol* 2002; **90**:631–633.

13.   Kandzari DE, Roe MT, Ohman EM, *et al*. Frequency, predictors, and outcomes of drug-eluting stent utilization in patients with high-risk non-ST-segment elevation acute coronary syndromes. *Am J Cardiol* 2005; **96**:750–755.

14.   Babapulle MN, Joseph L, Belisle P, *et al*. A hierarchical Bayesian meta-analysis of randomised clinical trials of drug-eluting stents. *Lancet* 2004; **364**:583–591.

15.   Bavry AA, Kumbhani DJ, Helton TJ, *et al*. Late thrombosis of drug-eluting stents: a meta-analysis of randomized clinical trials. *Am J Med* 2006; **119**:1056–1061.

16.   Stone GW, Moses JW, Ellis SG, *et al.* Safety and efficacy of sirolimus- and paclitaxel-eluting coronary stents. *N Engl J Med* 2007; **356**:998–1008.

17.   Bavry AA, Bhatt DL. Drug-eluting stents: dual anti-platelet therapy for every survivor? *Circulation* 2007; **116**:696–699.

18.   Spertus JA, Kettelkamp R, Vance C, *et al.* Prevalence, predictors, and outcomes of premature discontinuation of thienopyridine therapy after drug-eluting stent placement: results from the PREMIER registry. *Circulation* 2006; **113**:2803–2089.

19.   Bavry AA, Bhatt DL. Acute myocardial infarction and drug eluting stents: A green light for their use or time for measured restraint? *Am Heart J* 2007; **153**:719–721.

20.   Bavry AA, Bhatt DL. Appropriate use of drug-eluting stents: balancing the reduction in restenosis with the concern of late thrombosis. *Lancet* 2008; **371**:2134–43.

21.   OASIS-5 Trial Group. Comparison of fondaparinux and enoxaparin in acute coronary syndromes. *N Engl J Med* 2006; **354**:1464–1476.

22.   Yusuf S, Mehta SR, Chrolavicius S, *et al.*; for the OASIS-G Trial Group. Effects of fondaparinux on mortality and reinfarction in patients with acute ST-segment elevation myocardial infarction: the OASIS-6 randomized trial. *JAMA* 2006; 295:1519–1530.

23.   Cohen M, Bhatt DL, Alexander JH. Randomized, double-blind, dose-ranging study of otamixaban, a novel, parenteral, short-acting direct Factor Xa inhibitor, in percutaneous coronary intervention. The SEPIA-PCI Trial. *Circulation* 2007; **115**:2642–2651.

24.   Rajagopal V, Bhatt DL. Factor Xa inhibitors in acute coronary syndromes: moving from mythology to reality. *J Thromb Haemost* 2005; **3**:436–438.

25.   Meadows TA, Bhatt DL. Clinical aspects of platelet inhibitors and thrombus formation. *Circ Res* 2007; **100**:1261–1275.

26.   Canon CP, Husted S, Harrington RA, *et al.* Safety, tolerability, and initial efficacy of AZD6140, the first reversible oral adenosine diphosphate receptor antagonist, compared with clopidogrel, in patients with non-ST-segment elevation acute coronary syndrome: primary results of the DISPERSE-2 trial. *J Am Coll Cardiol* 2007; **50**:1844–1851.

27.   Limkakeng AT, Halpern E, Takakuwa KM. Sixty-four slice multidetector computed tomography: the future of ED cardiac care. *Am J Emerg Med* 2007; **25**:450–458.

Appendix:
ACC/AHA and ESC practice guidelines

Definitions for guideline recommendations and level of evidence	
Recommendation	**Definition**
Class I	Benefit markedly exceeds risk; therefore, the therapy should be performed
Class IIa	Benefit exceeds risk; therefore, it is reasonable to perform the therapy
Class IIb	Benefit may marginally exceed risk; therefore, the therapy can be performed under certain circumstances
Class III	Risk exceeds benefit; therefore, the therapy should not be performed
Level of evidence	**Definition**
Level A	Multiple studies with general consistency of direction and magnitude of treatment effect
Level B	Limited studies with less consistency of direction and magnitude of treatment effect
Level C	Very limited studies

Early invasive therapy versus conservative management

	ACC/AHA	ESC
Early invasive therapy is indicated for refractory angina, hemodynamic, or electrical instability (*urgent invasive therapy*)	I, B	I, C
Early invasive strategy is indicated in initially stabilized patients (without serious co-morbidities or contraindications) who have an elevated risk of clinical events (*semi-urgent invasive therapy; within 72 hours*)* • High risk score • Recurrent angina/ischemia at rest or low-level activities • Hemodynamic instability • Sustained ventricular tachycardia • Elevated cardiac biomarkers • New/presumably new ST-segment depression • Signs or symptoms of heart failure or new/worsening mitral regurgitation • High-risk findings from noninvasive testing • Percutaneous coronary intervention within 6 months • Prior coronary artery bypass grafting • Left ventricular ejection fraction ≤0.40	I, A	I, A
Initial conservative strategy can be considered in patients (without serious co-morbidities or contraindications to angiography) who have an elevated risk for clinical events, including troponin-positive patients, according to patient and physician preferences	IIb, B	
• A conservative strategy is recommended in women with low risk features	I, B	I, B[†]
Consideration should be given to the type of stent used (i.e., bare-metal versus drug-eluting)		I, C

*Additional ESC predictors of increased risk include diabetes mellitus, renal insufficiency, or an intermediate-to-high risk score. [†]The European Society of Cardiology (ESC) states that women should be evaluated and treated in the same way as men, with special attention to co-morbidities (I, B). ACC, American College of Cardiology; AHA, American Heart Association.

Adjunctive anti-platelet and anti-coagulation therapies – invasive strategy

	ACC/AHA	ESC
Initiate aspirin (or clopidogrel if intolerant) as soon as possible after presentation	I, A	I, A
• Bare-metal stent:		
• Aspirin 162–325 mg/day for at least 1 month, then 75–162 mg/day indefinitely	I, A	I, A[†]
• Clopidogrel 75 mg/day for at least 1 month	I, A	
• Clopidogrel 75 mg/day for up to 1 year	I, B	I, A
• Drug-eluting stent:		
• Aspirin 162–325 mg/day for at least 3 months (sirolimus) to 6 months (paclitaxel), then 75–162 mg/day indefinitely	I, A	I, A[†]
• Clopidogrel 75 mg/day for at least 1 year	I, B	I, A
Initiate anti-coagulant therapy as soon as possible after presentation*	I, A	I, A
• Unfractionated heparin	I, A	I, C
• Enoxaparin	I, A	IIa, B
• Bivalirudin	I, B	I, B
• Fondaparinux	I, B	I, A[‡]
Prior to angiography, initiate either clopidogrel or a glycoprotein IIb/IIIa inhibitor	I, A	
A glycoprotein IIb/IIIa inhibitor must be combined with an anticoagulant		I, A
Clopidogrel and eptifibitide or tirofiban can be used prior to angiography if:	IIa, B	IIa, A
• Delay to angiography		
• High risk features		
• Early recurrent ischemic symptoms		
In high-risk patients not pretreated with a glycoprotein IIb/IIIa inhibitor and proceeding to intervention, abciximab is recommended immediately following angiography		I, A

*Anti-coagulation can be terminated after revascularization unless there is a compelling indication for its ongoing use. [†]The European Society of Cardiology (ESC) dose for chronic aspirin is 75–100 mg/day. [‡]The ESC states that as long as a decision is being considered between an invasive versus a conservative strategy, the use of fonda-parinux is recommended. See Appendix III for recommendations on adjunctive medical therapies. ACC, American College of Cardiology; AHA, American Heart Association.

Adjunctive anti-platelet, anti-coagulation, medical therapies, and risk stratification – conservative strategy

	ACC/AHA	ESC
Initiate aspirin (or clopidogrel if intolerant) as soon as possible after presentation	I, A	I, A
• Aspirin 75–162 mg/day indefinitely	I, A	
• Aspirin 75–100 mg/day indefinitely		I, A
Initiate clopidogrel loading (300–600 mg) and maintenance dose in addition to aspirin	I, A	
• Clopidogrel 75 mg/day at least 1 month	I, A	
• Clopidogrel 75 mg/day for up to 1 year	I, B	I, A
Patients pre-treated with clopidogrel who later need surgical revascularization should have clopidogrel held for at least 5 days	I, B*	IIa, C
Eptifibitide or tirofiban can be added to aspirin and clopidogrel if high risk features	IIb, B	
Initiate anti-coagulant therapy as soon as possible after presentation[†,‡]	I, A	I, A
• Unfractionated heparin	I, A	
• Enoxaparin (may be preferable)	I, A	IIa, B
• Bivalirudin		
• Fondaparinux (may be preferable)	I, B	I, A
ACE inhibitor		
• Initiate oral therapy within 24 hours with pulmonary congestion or left ventricular ejection fraction ≤0.40, in absence of hypotension (systolic blood pressure <100 mmHg)	I, A	I, A[§]
• Angiotensin receptor blocker if ACE inhibitor intolerant	I, A	I, B
• Can be given to patients without pulmonary congestion or left ventricular dysfunction	IIa, B	IIa, B
• Intravenous therapy in first 24 hours may be harmful	III, B	
Beta blocker therapy	I, B	I, B
• Initiate oral therapy within first 24 hours unless heart failure, low-output state, increased risk for cardiogenic shock, or relative contraindications		I, A
• Should be given to all patients with reduced left ventricular function	IIa, B	
• Intravenous therapy for high blood pressure without contraindications	III, A	
• Intravenous therapy if signs of heart failure, low-output state, or other risk factors for cardiogenic shock		

Adjunctive anti-platelet, anti-coagulation, medical therapies, and risk stratification – conservative strategy *Continued*

	ACC/AHA	ESC
Lipid management		
• Statin (in absence of contraindications) should be given regardless of baseline LDL cholesterol during hospitalization	I, A	I, B
• Fasting lipid profile within 24 hours		
• Goal LDL:	I, C	
<100 mg/dL		
<70 mg/dL reasonable	I, A	
• Triglycerides and non-HDL cholesterol:	IIa, A	IIa, B
• If triglycerides 200–499 mg/dL, non-HDL-C should be <130 mg/dL		
• Triglycerides ≥500 mg/dL, fibrate or niacin should be started before LDL-C lowering to prevent pancreatitis	I, B I, C	
Aldosterone receptor blockade should be prescribed long term if there is no significant renal dysfunction or hyperkalemia and if the patient is already on an ACE inhibitor, with left ventricular ejection fraction ≤0.40, and either symptomatic heart failure or diabetes	I, A	I, B
A stress test should be performed during hospitalization for assessment of ischemia	I, B	I, C
• If the patient is classified as not low risk, diagnostic angiography should be performed	I, A	
• If left ventricular ejection fraction is ≤0.40, it is reasonable to perform diagnostic angiography	IIa, B	
Blood pressure control		
• <140/90 mmHg	I, A	
• <130/80 mmHg with diabetes mellitus or chronic kidney disease	I, A	
Smoking cessation and avoidance of exposure to environmental tobacco	I, B	
NSAIDs and COX-2-selective agents:		
• Discontinue at hospital presentation	I, C	
• NSAIDs and COX-2 inhibitors should not be used with aspirin or clopidogrel		III, C
• At discharge, treat chronic musculoskeletal pain relief with acetaminophen, small-dose narcotics, or nonacetylated salicylates	I, A	
• Naproxen may be reasonable if above insufficient	IIa, C	

Adjunctive anti-platelet, anti-coagulation, medical therapies, and risk stratification – conservative strategy *Continued*

	ACC/AHA	ESC
Miscellaneous:		
• Cardiac rehabilitation	I, C	
• Menopausal hormone therapy should not be given for secondary prevention of coronary events	III, A	
• Antioxidant vitamin supplements (C, E, or beta-carotene) and folic acid (with or without B_6 and B_{12}) should not be used for secondary prevention	III, A	

*Surgery can be performed more urgently than 5 days if the increased bleeding risk is considered acceptable (class IC). †If the decision is made to perform percutaneous coronary intervention, the initial anti-coagulant should be maintained during the procedure, except for fondaparinux where additional unfractionated heparin (50 units/kg bolus) should be given. ‡Anti-coagulation can be maintained until hospital discharge if there is no bleeding. §European Society of Cardiology (ESC) includes diabetes, hypertension, or chronic kidney disease as class Ia recommendations for use of an angiotensin-converting enzyme (ACE) inhibitor. ACC, American College of Cardiology; AHA, American Heart Association; COX, cyclooxygenase; HDL, high-density lipoprotein; LDL, low-density lipoprotein; NSAID, nonsteroidal anti-inflammatory drug.

Index

Page references to *figures, tables and text boxes* are shown in *italics*.

Registries, studies and trials have been indexed under their acronyms/abbreviations and have been grouped together.

abciximab anti-platelet
  therapy, 27
  dosage recommendations, 41–2
ACC/AHA and ESC practice
  guidelines
  adjunctive anti-platelet,
    anticoagulation, medical
    therapies, and risk
    stratification, conservative
    strategy, *71*
  adjunctive anti-platelet and anti
    coagulation therapies, invasive
    strategy *79*
  early invasive therapy
    vs. conservative management,
    80
  levels of evidence, 80
ACE inhibitors 61
Acute coronary syndromes
  Definition, 1
  mortality 3–4, *6*
  pathogenesis, inflammation in, 62
  prognosis, 3
  see also cardiovascular disease
ADP receptor inhibitors, 40
Angina 15–16
angiotensin receptor blockers, 62
angiotensin-converting enzyme
  inhibitors, 62
anti-coagulants *see* anti-thrombin
  therapy

anti-platelet therapy40
  ACC/AHA and ESC practice
    guidelines, 30
  benefits by patient subgroup, *41*
anti-thrombin therapy, 49–57
  ACC/AHA and ESC practice
    guidelines, 30
Aspirin
  anti-platelet therapy, 37–45
  coagulation cascade blocking, 14
  dosage recommendations, 38
  ibuprofen interaction, 38
  incidence of major bleeding, 38,
    43, 79
  plus clopidogrel, 39–41, *43,* 52
atherosclerosis
  pathophysiology, 11–13
  risk factors, 11
atorvastatin, 61
AZD 6140, 85

bare-metal stents *vs.* drug-eluting
  stents, 81–85
beta-blockers, 63–65
  in low-risk acute myocardial
    infarction, *64*
biomarkers, 16–18
bivalirudin
  anti-thrombin agent, 49–51
  dosage recommendation, 56
  vs. GPIIb/IIIa inhibitor, *56*
  vs. heparin, *55*

blood pressure, 5

calcified nodule, *13*
calcium-channel blockers, 64
cangrelor, 85
captopril, 62
cardiovascular disease
  age and gender factors, 29
  incidence, 2
  prevalence and overlap of
      forms 2
    see also acute coronary
        syndromes
  clinical manifestations, 15–21
clopidogrel
  anti-platelet therapy, 40, 82–83
  with aspirin 39–40
  dosage recommendations, 41
  structure   *42*
coagulation cascade, 14
computed tomography, 64-slice
    multi-detector, 86
culprit-vessel *vs.* multi-vessel
    intervention, 81

diabetes, 5
direct thrombin inhibitors, 54–57
  dosage recommendations, 56
dosage recommendations
  abciximab, 43, 44
  aspirin, 37–40
  bivalirudin, 55
  clopidogrel, 41
  direct thrombin inhibitors, 55
  factor Xa inhibitors, 57
  fondaparinux, 55
  glycoprotein IIb/IIIa inhibitors,
      42–45

low-molecular-weight heparin
    (LMWH), 51–54
  unfractionated heparin (UFH),
      49–51
drug-eluting stents, 40, 74
  vs. bare-metal stents, 81–85

electrocardiogram (ECG), 18–21, *26*
enoxaparin, 49, *52*
  anti-thrombin agent, 49–51
  vs. unfractionated heparin (UFH),
      49–51, *52, 53*

facilitated percutaneous coronary
    intervention, 75, 79
factor Xa inhibitors
  anti-thrombin agents, 49
  dosage recommendation, 57
  vs. LMWH 57
fondaparinux
  anti-thrombin agents, 49
  dosage recommendation, 57

glycoprotein IIb/IIIa inhibitors
  anti-platelet therapies, 37–45
  coagulation cascade blocking, 14
  dosage recommendations, 44–45
  intravenous *vs.* oral, 64
  major bleeding increase, 38, 43, 44
  pre cardiac catheterization, 44
  vs. bivalirudin, 54, *55*
GRACE (Global Registry of Acute
    Coronary Events) risk
    score, 28, *32*
  patient management *32*

heparin *see* low-molecular-
    weight heparin (LMWH);
    unfractionated heparin (UFH)
heparin-induced
    thrombocytopenia, 51
HMG-CoA reductase inhibitors *see*
    statins

ibuprofen, interaction with aspirin,
    38

lesions, stenotic *vs.* non-stenotic *12*
low-molecular-weight heparin
    (LMWH)
  anti-thrombin agent, 51–54
  dosage recommendations, 54
  vs. unfractionated heparin (UFH),
    54

metoprolol, 64
multi-vessel intervention *vs.*
    culprit-vessel, 81
myocardial infarction
  odds ratios and scoring system *21*
  see also non-ST-elevation;
    ST-elevation

nitrates, as anti-anginal agents, 64
nitroglycerin, angina relief 16
non-ST-elevation myocardial
    infarction
  biomarkers, 16–18
  definition, 12
  pharmacological management,
    guideline recommended
    therapy use, 9
  revascularization and intervention
    therapy, 69–75

guideline recommended therapy
    use, *9*
risk models, 24–34
  see also ST-elevation, guideline
    recommended therapy use

pathophysiology 11–14
physical inactivity, prevalence, 5
plaque rupture, 11–13
  spontaneous healing 12
platelet activation and aggregation
    in ischemic syndromes, *42*
prasugrel, 40–41
  structure, 41
prognosis determination *see* risk
    stratification
PURSUIT risk score, 25, 26, *29*

ranolazine 65
registries, studies and trials
  ACUITY timing trial *43*, 44, 54
  Anti-Platelet Trialists'
    Collaboration 37
  CAPRIE trial 39–40
  COMMIT trial 40, 64–5
  CREATE study 53
  CRUSADE registry 30–1
  CURE trial 38, 39–40
  ESSENCE trial 24
  ExTRACT trial 54
  FINESSE trial 44, 79
  GRACE Registry 4, *25*, 28–30
  GUSTO-1 trial 33
  ICTUS trial 72–4, 80
  MIRACL trial 61
  OASIS trial 55–6
  PROVE-IT trial 61

PURSUIT trial 27–30
SYNERGY study 52
TACTICS-TIMI 18 trial 30, 70, 72
TARGET trial 44
TRITON-TIMI 38 trial 41
VANQWISH trial 69–71
reperfusion therapy 75
revascularization therapy 69–74
  angiography 74
  invasive *vs.* conservative strategies 71, 80
  guidelines 84
  probability of event-free survival 70
risk stratification 23–35
  in-hospital mortality 30, 32
  troponin status 71, 72

smoking, prevalence 5
statins 61–63
  in ACS pathogenesis 63
  cardiovascular outcomes in statin therapy 62
ST-elevation myocardial infarction
  definition 12
  guideline recommended therapy use
    pharmacological management 6
    reperfusion and intervention therapy 9
  risk models 24, 31–34
  see also non-ST-elevation
stenting
  benefit maximization algorithm 83, 84

culprit-vessel *versus* multi-vessel intervention 81
drug-eluting stents 74
drug-eluting stents *vs.* bare-metal stents 81–83
safety and efficacy optimization algorithm85
ST-segment elevation, biomarkers 16–18, 17
substernal chest heaviness 16
symptoms and signs 15–16

T value elevation , 17
thienopyridines, coagulation cascade blocking 14
TIMI (Thrombolysis in Myocardial Infarction) risk score 24–30, 25, 26, 27, 28, 30, 33, 56, 71, 72
  STEMI 30-day mortality 32
troponin status 17, 17, 56, 71, 72, 73, 81

unfractionated heparin (UFH)
  anti-thrombin agent 49
  benefits 50, 52
  dosage recommendations 51
  side effects 86
  vs. enoxaparin 49, 51, 52, 53–54, 55, 56–57
  vs. low-molecular-weight heparin (LMWH) 51–54
unstable coronary event, causes 12, 13

World Heath Organization (WHO), mortality statistics 2

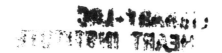

Printed in the United States